ABC OF RESUSCITATION

ABC OF RESUSCITATION

edited by

MICHAEL COLQUHOUN
General practitioner, Malvern

ANTHONY J HANDLEY
Consultant physician and cardiologist,
Colchester General Hospital, Colchester

T R EVANS
Consultant cardiologist,
Royal Free Hospital, London

on behalf of
the Resuscitation Council (UK)
with contributions from the
following members of the Resuscitation Council

PETER J F BASKETT, A JOHN CAMM, DOUGLAS CHAMBERLAIN,
T R EVANS, JUDITH M FISHER, MARK HARRIES,
ANDREW K MARSDEN, A D MILNER, ANTHONY D REDMOND,
R S SIMONS, BRIAN STEGGLES, ANDREW H SWAIN,
RICHARD VINCENT, DAVID A ZIDEMAN

and additional contributions from
G A D REES, B A WILLIS, GERALYN WYNNE

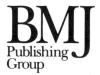

First published in 1986
by the BMJ Publishing Group, BMA House, Tavistock Square,
London WC1H 9JR

First edition 1986
Second impression 1988
Third impression 1988
Fourth impression 1989
Second edition 1990
Second impression 1991
Third impression 1992
Third edition 1995

British Library Cataloguing in Publication Data

A catalogue record for this book is available from the
British Library

ISBN 0-7279-0839-1

Typeset by Apek Typesetters Ltd., Nailsea, Bristol
Printed in Great Britain by Eyre & Spottiswoode Ltd, Margate

Contents

INTRODUCTION

During the 1950s the work of researchers like Elam, Safer, and Gordon established expired air ventilation (the kiss of life or mouth to mouth respiration) as the most effective method of providing artificial ventilation for a casualty who has stopped breathing. In 1960 Jude, Kouwenhoven, and Knickerbocker published their classic work on closed chest cardiac compression, showing that the circulation could be maintained during cardiac arrest without the need for thoracotomy. Closed chest defibrillation came into widespread use at the same time, making the successful resuscitation of patients with ventricular fibrillation a common occurrence in hospital.

Special units where prompt resuscitation was available to patients at high risk of developing cardiac arrest became part of routine hospital practice. Thus coronary care units for patients with acute myocardial infarction were established, with the realisation that most deaths from the condition occurred in the early stages, not because the myocardium was severely damaged but because of potentially treatable disturbance in rhythm.

Once the effectiveness of resuscitation in hospital became established, the realisation that two thirds of deaths from coronary heart disease occurred before hospital admission led to attempts to provide coronary care, and particularly defibrillation, in the community. The credit for this goes to Pantridge in Belfast, who pioneered the first mobile coronary care unit staffed by a doctor and a nurse. Their early experience confirmed the high incidence of lethal arrhythmias at the onset of myocardial infarction, and many patients attended by his mobile units were successfully resuscitated from cardiac arrest before admission to hospital. Pantridge and his coworkers also drew attention to the value of cardiopulmonary resuscitation performed by a bystander when cardiac arrest occurred before the arrival of the mobile unit.

In the early 1970s, Leonard Cobb, a cardiologist in Seattle, inspired by these results, equipped paramedics with defibrillators and also trained firefighters to perform basic life support. The fire service in Seattle is highly coordinated, and a standard fire appliance can reach any part of the city within four minutes so that cardiopulmonary resuscitation would already be in progress when more highly trained paramedics arrived in an ambulance some minutes later. The most crucial determinant of survival from cardiac arrest was found to be the speed with which defibrillation was performed. To accelerate this further the basic firefighters were equipped with defibrillators, a process facilitated by the development of the semiautomatic advisory model that requires less training to use.

Vickery, the chief of the fire service in Seattle, made the crucial suggestion that cardiopulmonary resuscitation by citizens might be the first stage in the provision of coronary care outside hospital. With Cobb he inaugurated training in resuscitation techniques for the public to increase further the practice of cardiopulmonary resuscitation. Research in Seattle and the surrounding area of King County has confirmed the importance of rapid institution of basic life support, together with early defibrillation, in determining survival from cardiac arrest occurring outside hospital. Intensive efforts to reduce delays to the minimum have resulted in survival rates of up to 40% being reported from that part of the United States.

In the United Kingdom progress in community resuscitation has been slower to gain momentum, but recently advances have been made. Scotland became the first country in the world to equip every emergency ambulance with a defibrillator, and these are now standard equipment nationwide. In the near future every front line ambulance will carry at least one trained paramedic. Already, survival rates of 50% have been reported after cardiac arrest witnessed by an ambulance crew. Many new initiatives to train the public in basic cardiopulmonary resuscitation are also being made; survival rates of around 15% have been reported when this takes place before the arrival of the ambulance.

We must not forget that hospital staff often do not possess even the basic resuscitation skills that might be expected. Several studies have shown alarmingly poor performance of resuscitation techniques by junior doctors and nurses and rapid decay in skills after tuition. The need for more extensive training in both basic and advanced life support, with regular practice and frequent revision, has become a priority in the training of medical and nursing staff. Further work is required to determine the best methods of training, the best manikins for practice, and the optimal frequency of training.

The Resuscitation Council (UK) comprises doctors from many different disciplines who share the desire to improve standards of resuscitation, both in hospital and in the community. Members of the council with other invited experts produced the first edition of the ABC in 1986, not as a manual or textbook but as a guide to resuscitation in the late 1980s. Our intention with this edition is to provide the same guide for the 1990s.

MICHAEL COLQUHOUN
ANTHONY J HANDLEY
T R EVANS

Resuscitation Council,
9 Fitzroy Square,
London W1P 5AH

1995

Introduction to the third edition

There have been many developments in resuscitation since the publication of the second edition of the ABC in 1990. Since that time the European Resuscitation Council has become established as the principal advisory body on the practice of resuscitation in Europe. Many of the key positions in the council are currently held by members of the Resuscitation Council (UK). The third edition of the ABC has been completely updated to incorporate the current European guidelines on the management of the three main types of cardiac arrest: ventricular fibrillation, asystole, and electromechanical dissociation. In October 1994 at the Second International Symposium of the European Resuscitation Council in Mainz, Germany, guidelines on the management of arrhythmias that precede cardiac arrest or complicate the early period after resuscitation were published. These have become known as the "peri-arrest arrhythmias", and their management forms the basis of a new chapter.

Major new initiatives in the training of resuscitation techniques have been introduced in the United Kingdom since 1990. The launch of Heartstart UK by the British Heart Foundation in 1992, with help from members of the Resuscitation Council (UK), marked a landmark in the training of members of the public in basic life support. Training in advanced life support techniques for members of the medical and allied professions have been standardised with the introduction of the Resuscitation Council's advanced life suppport course. Both these developments are described in an additional chapter on training and retention of skills.

New chapters have been added on the roles of cardiac pacing and drugs in the treatment of cardiac arrest. The chapter on resuscitation by the ambulance service has been completely revised in the light of the rapid advances in the training and equipment of ambulance crews that have taken place recently in this country. All other chapters have been revised, some very extensively, and we are grateful to the authors for the considerable amount of work they have devoted to this. Many new illustrations have been prepared and we are confident that these will enhance the value of this book.

The publication *ABC of Major Trauma* describes in detail the resuscitation of victims of trauma; it was therefore decided not to include the two previously published chapters on resuscitation in the accident and emergency department and resuscitation of multiply injured patients.

We hope that this edition will prove as popular as its predecessors and help everyone who treats the victims of sudden cardiac arrest to improve their management of a condition that remains a leading cause of death in the United Kingdom.

MICHAEL COLQUHOUN
Chairman of the research working party
Resuscitation Council (UK)

ANTHONY J HANDLEY
Secretary of the Resuscitation Council (UK)
Chairman of the basic life support working party
of the European Resuscitation Council

T R EVANS
Chairman of the advanced life support working party
Resuscitation Council (UK)

Acknowledgements

The editors are grateful to the following for help with illustrations of equipment:

Ambu International, Midsomer Norton, Bath; Cook Critical Care (UK); Laerdal Medical Ltd, Orpington, Kent; Physio Control Ltd, Basingstoke, Hampshire; Survivalink/Ferno (UK) Ltd, Bradford, West Yorkshire; Vitalograph Ltd, Maids Morton, Buckingham; Zoll Medical (UK) Ltd, Manchester.

The line diagram of a laryngeal mask airway on p 24 is redrawn from *General Surgical Operations* (RM Kirk, ed) and reproduced with permission of Churchill Livingstone.

We thank many people, particularly Liz Bruce and staff at Worcester Royal Infirmary, for help with other illustrations. We also thank Jim and Ann Silk for help preparing many of the photographic illustrations, and Linda Norman for considerable secretarial help.

1 BASIC LIFE SUPPORT

Judith M Fisher, Anthony J Handley

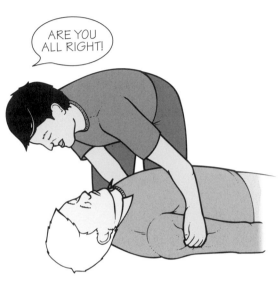

Basic life support means the maintenance of an airway and the support of breathing and the circulation without the use of equipment other than a simple airway device or protective shield. A combination of expired air ventilation and chest compression is known as cardiopulmonary resuscitation and forms the basis of modern basic life support. The term "cardiac arrest" implies a sudden interruption of cardiac output which may be reversible with appropriate treatment. It does not include the cessation of heart activity as a terminal event in serious illness; in these circumstances the techniques of basic life support are usually inappropriate.

Survival from cardiac arrest is most likely when the event is witnessed; when a bystander summons help from the emergency services and starts resuscitation; when the heart arrests in ventricular fibrillation; and when defibrillation and advanced life support are instituted at an early stage. Basic life support is one link in this chain of survival.

Basic life support is the emergency treatment of any condition in which the brain suddenly fails to receive enough oxygen. It involves assessment followed by action—the ABC: A is for assessment and airway; B is for breathing; C is for circulation.

Assessment

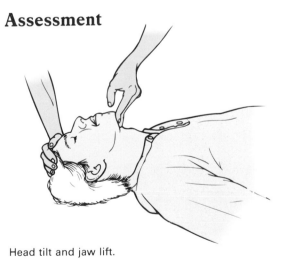

Head tilt and jaw lift.

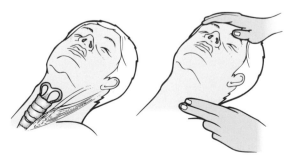

Rapidly assess any danger to the casualty and yourself from such hazards as falling masonry, gas, electricity, fire, or traffic; there is no sense in having two casualties. Establish whether the casualty is responsive by gently shaking his or her shoulders and asking loudly "Are you all right?" Be careful not to aggravate any existing injury, particularly of the cervical spine.

If there is no response shout for help or send a bystander to telephone for an ambulance. Complete your assessment by opening the airway, checking for breathing, and checking the pulse.

Establishing and maintaining an airway is the single most useful manoeuvre the rescuer can perform and is a necessary prerequisite to completing your assessment of the casualty.

Loosen tight clothing around the casualty's neck and remove any obvious obstruction from the mouth; leave well fitting dentures in place. Extend, but do not hyperextend, the neck thus lifting the tongue off the posterior wall of the pharynx. This is best achieved by placing your hand along the casualty's upper forehead and exerting pressure to tilt the head, at the same time placing two fingertips under the point of the chin to lift it forwards. This will often allow breathing to restart.

Look, listen, and feel for breathing: *look* for chest movement; *listen* close to the mouth for breath sounds; and *feel* for air with your cheek. Look, listen, and feel for five seconds before deciding that breathing is absent.

Check for a pulse. The best pulse to feel in an emergency is the carotid, but if the neck is injured the pulse may be felt at the femoral artery. Feel for five seconds before deciding it is absent.

1

Action

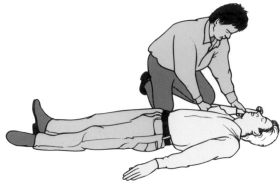

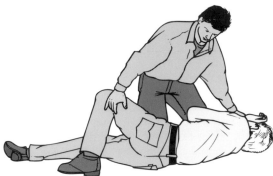

Turning casualty to recovery position.

Recovery position

If the casualty is unconscious but has a pulse and is breathing place him or her in the recovery position, if necessary supporting the chin to maintain an airway. In this position the tongue will fall away from the pharyngeal wall and any vomit or secretion will dribble out of the corner of the mouth rather than obstruct the airway or, later on, cause aspiration pneumonia.

Go or telephone for help if your initial call has not been answered.

If the pulse or breathing is absent your subsequent action should again follow the ABC: airway; breathing; circulation.

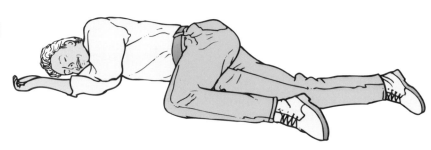

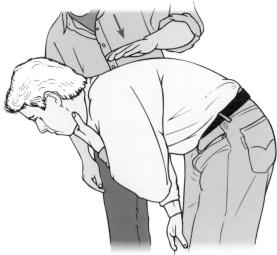

Choking and back blows.

Airway

If after tilting the head and lifting the chin the airway still seems to be obstructed there may be a foreign body present. First try to remove this by finger sweeps in the mouth. If this is not successful give five firm back blows between the scapulae; this may dislodge a foreign body by compressing the air that remains in the lungs thereby producing an upward force behind the obstructing material.

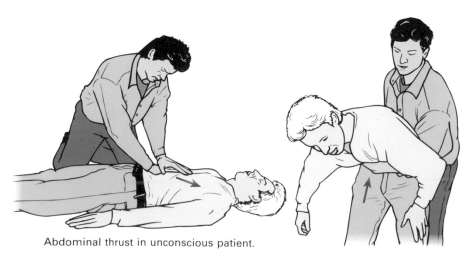

Abdominal thrust in unconscious patient.

If both finger sweeps and back blows fail to clear the airway try five abdominal thrusts. In an unconscious person kneel over the casualty, make a fist of one of your hands and place it immediately below the casualty's xiphisternum.

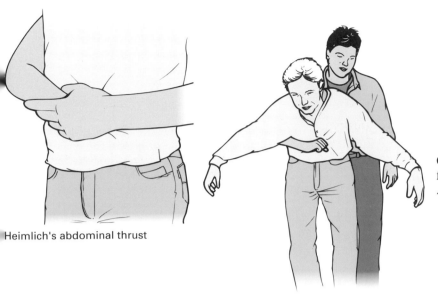

Grasp this fist with your other hand and push firmly and suddenly upwards and posteriorly. Alternate abdominal thrusts with back slaps.

Heimlich's abdominal thrust

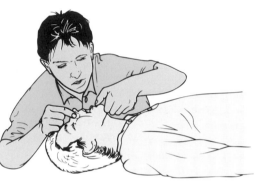

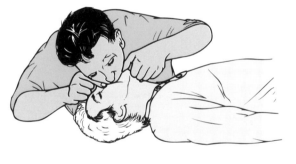

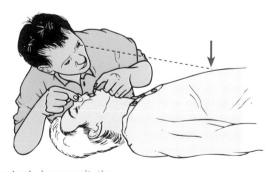

Expired air resuscitation.

Breathing

If there is no breathing but a pulse is present make certain the casualty is on his or her back and give 10 breaths of expired air ventilation. Maintain an airway by tilting the head and lifting the chin. Pinch closed the nose with the fingers of your hand on the forehead. Take a deep breath, seal your lips firmly around those of the casualty, and breathe out until you see the casualty's chest clearly rising, taking about two seconds for a full ventilation. Lift your head away, watching the casualty's chest fall, and take another breath of air; the chest should rise as you blow in and fall when you take your mouth away. Each breath should visibly expand the casualty's chest but not cause over inflation as this will allow air to enter the oesophagus and stomach. Subsequent gastric distention not only causes vomiting but passive regurgitation into the lungs which often goes undetected. After 10 ventilations, if the casualty is still not breathing and help is not on its way, go and telephone for an ambulance. Return to the casualty, reassess consciousness, breathing, and the pulse and continue ventilation as necessary, rechecking the pulse after every 10 breaths.

Circulation

If the pulse is absent (cardiac arrest) it is unlikely that the casualty will recover as a result of cardiopulmonary resuscitation alone; defibrillation and other advanced life support is urgently required. If your initial calls for help have produced no response and no one else is

> **If no breathing and no pulse telephone for help immediately**

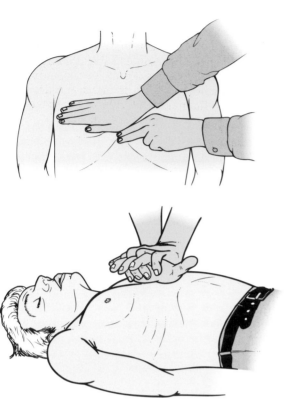

available you should leave the casualty at this point and go yourself to telephone for an ambulance. On your return ensure that the casualty is on his or her back on a firm, flat surface. Open the airway by tilting the head and lifting the chin and give two breaths of expired air ventilation. Then start chest compressions.

The correct place to compress is in the centre of the lower half of the sternum. To find this, and to ensure that the risk of damaging intra-abdominal organs is minimised, feel along the rib margin until you come to the xiphisternum; place your middle finger on the xiphisternum and your index finger on the bony sternum above. Slide the heel of your other hand down to these fingers and leave it there. Remove your first hand and place it on top of the second. Press down firmly keeping your arms straight and elbows locked. In an adult compress about 4–5 cm keeping the pressure firm, controlled, and applied vertically. Try to spend about the same time in the compressed phase as in the released phase and aim for a rate of 80 compressions a minute.

After each 15 compressions tilt the head, lift the chin, and give two inflations. Return your hands immediately to the sternum and give 15 further compressions continuing compressions and ventilations in a ratio of 15:2. It may help to get the right rate and ratio by counting: "One and two and three . . ."

If two trained rescuers are present one should assume responsibility for ventilation and the other for chest compression. The compression rate should remain at 80 per minute, but there should be a pause after each five compressions just long enough to allow a single ventilation to be given over about two seconds. Provided the casualty's airway is maintained it is not necessary to wait for exhalation before resuming chest compressions.

Precordial thump

There is evidence that an initial precordial (chest) thump may restart the recently arrested heart. This is particularly the case if the onset of cardiac arrest is witnessed on an electrocardiograph monitor. For this reason the precordial thump is taught as a standard part of advanced life support.

Dangers of resuscitation

Until fairly recently the main concern in resuscitation was for the casualty but attention has now been directed towards the rescuer, particularly in the light of fears about the transmission of AIDS. No case of AIDS, however, has yet been reported due to transfer from casualty to rescuer (or vice versa) by mouth to mouth resuscitation. Despite the presence of the virus in saliva it does not seem that transmission occurs via this route in the absence of blood to blood contact. Nevertheless, there is still an understandable concern about the possible risk of infection, and those who may be called on to administer resuscitation should be allowed the use of some form of barrier device. This may take the form of a ventilation mask (for mouth to mask ventilation) or a filter device placed over the mouth and nose. The main requirement of these devices is that they should not hinder an adequate flow of air and not provide too great a dead space. Resuscitation must not be delayed while such a device is being sought.

Future developments

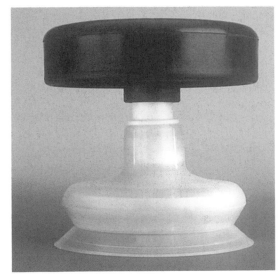

Active compression and decompression device.

Active compression-decompression resuscitation is a technique of cardiopulmonary resuscitation that employs a hand held suction device applied to the lower sternum. It is used to compress the chest at the same rate as in normal cardiopulmonary resuscitation, but after each compression phase it is actively lifted, the suction cup maintaining contact with the skin. This enhances decompression of the thorax and in studies on animals and humans has been shown to increase venous return and left ventricular filling. Preliminary studies have suggested that this is a simple technique which may improve outcome after cardiac arrest.

Further reading

Tucker KJ, Idris A. Clinical and laboratory investigations of active compression-decompression cardiopulmonary resuscitation. *Resuscitation* 1994; **28**: 1–7.

Lurie KG. Active compression-decompression CPR: a progress report. *Resuscitation* 1994; **28**: 115–122.

European Resuscitation Council Basic Life Support Working Group. Guidelines for basic life support. *BMJ* 1993; **306**: 1587–9.

2 VENTRICULAR FIBRILLATION

Michael Colquhoun, Douglas Chamberlain

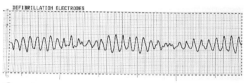

Onset.

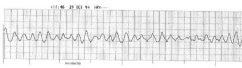

Five minutes.

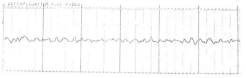

Ten minutes.

The amplitude of ventricular fibrillation becomes progressively smaller with time.

The normal cardiac cycle is controlled by an orderly sequence of depolarisation spreading through specialised conducting tissue to the ventricular myocardium. In ventricular fibrillation this orderly sequence is lost and individual cardiac muscle cells depolarise in a chaotic fashion; all coordinated muscular activity is lost, resulting in cardiac arrest. In the absence of coronary flow the myocardium becomes progressively more ischaemic, and irreversible cerebral anoxic damage occurs within a very few minutes. Coronary perfusion also falls to zero during ventricular fibrillation with the result that progressive ischaemia occurs throughout the myocardium.

The definitive treatment of ventricular fibrillation is the application of a defibrillatory electrical countershock. The sooner this can be given after the onset of ventricular fibrillation the greater the chance of success. In the absence of defibrillation the amplitude of the fibrillatory wave form progressively decreases until terminal asystole supervenes; this process is slowed by effective basic life support.

Epidemiology

> **All GPs and ambulance staff, who provide initial treatment, should have the equipment and skills to defibrillate**

Ventricular fibrillation is the commonest mode of cardiac arrest, particularly in patients with ischaemic heart disease. It is far more likely to respond to treatment than asystole or electromechanical dissociation, which are considered in chapter 3. Ventricular fibrillation (which may be preceeded by ventricular tachycardia) is seen in up to 80–90% of patients dying suddenly outside hospital. It is particularly common in the early stages of myocardial infarction, which emphasises the importance of general practitioners and ambulance staff, who provide the initial medical treatment for these patients, having the equipment and ability to defibrillate.

Electrocardiographic appearances

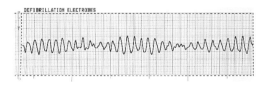

The electrocardiogram shows a bizarre irregular wave form apparently random in both frequency and amplitude. Ventricular fibrillation is sometimes classified as either coarse or fine depending on the amplitude of the complexes. The treatment of both forms is identical. The only practical implications of this distinction are to give some indication of the potential for successful defibrillation and to serve as a reminder that fine ventricular fibrillation may be mistaken for asystole.

Electrical defibrillation

The definitive treatment of ventricular fibrillation is the application of a defibrillatory countershock; only rarely will it remit spontaneously, and no drug has been shown to have a useful defibrillation effect. A precordial thump may on occasions abolish the arrhythmia when applied very soon after its onset and should be considered in cases of witnessed, particularly monitored, cardiac arrest.

Defibrillation aims to depolarise most of the myocardium simultaneously, allowing the natural pacemaking tissues to resume control of the heart. Successful defibrillation will follow depolarisation of a critical mass of myocardium; this in turn depends on the actual current flow (measured in amperes) rather than the energy of the delivered shock (measured in joules). The magnitude of current flow is a function of transthoracic impedance, body size, electrode position, and the energy of the shock delivered.

Transthoracic impedance

The magnitude of the current passing through the heart will depend on the voltage delivered by the defibrillator and the impedance to current flow through the chest wall, lungs, and myocardium (the transthoracic impedance). Transthoracic impedance is influenced by the size of the electrodes and the interface between these and the skin; the usual electrode sizes are 10–13 cm for adults and 4.5–8 cm for infants and children. Impedance between the electrodes and the skin is minimised by the use of conductive electrode gel or defibrillator pads. Impedance may be minimised by applying firm pressure to the electrode paddles to maintain optimal skin contact; this is at its least when the lungs are empty so defibrillation is best carried out in the expiratory phase of ventilation.

Body size

Infants and children require shocks of less energy to achieve defibrillation than adults. Over the usual range of weight encountered in adults, however, body size does not greatly influence energy requirements.

Electrode position

The ideal electrode position is one that allows maximum current to flow through the myocardium. The standard technique is to place one electrode to the right of the upper part of the sternum below the clavicle and the other in the fifth left intercostal space in the mid-clavicular to the anterior axillary line, the position corresponding to the cardiac apex or V4/V5 of the electrocardiogram. An alternative, which may be tried if initial attempts at defibrillation are unsuccessful, is to place one electrode to the left of the lower sternal border and the other on the posterior chest wall below the left scapula.

Special care is required when the patient has an implanted pacemaker. Current may travel down the electrode of the pacemaker and cause burns at the site where the tip of the electrode lies against the myocardium. This may lead to a considerable rise in the threshold of pacing which may become apparent only a considerable time later. To minimise this risk the defibrillator electrodes should be placed at least 12·5 cm from the pacemaker unit. If resuscitation is successful, regular checks on the threshold of the pacemaker should be carried out over the following two months.

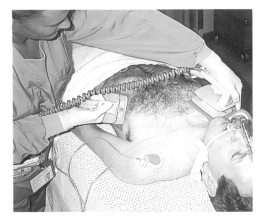

Electrode positions for manual defibrillation.

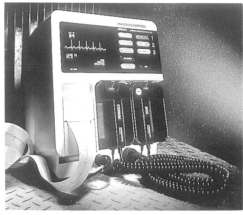

Manual defibrillator.

Defibrillators

Electrical energy from rechargeable batteries or from the mains is used to charge a capacitor, and the energy stored is subsequently discharged through electrodes placed on the casualty's chest. The energy stored in the capacitor may be varied by a manual control, the calibration points on which represent the delivered energy measured in joules(J). 200J and 360J are the usual energy levels used in the treatment of ventricular fibrillation.

Modern defibrillators allow monitoring of the electrocardiogram through the defibrillator electrodes and display the rhythm on a screen. With a manual defibrillator the operator interprets the rhythm and decides if a defibrillatory countershock is indicated. The strength of the shock is set manually, the capacitor is charged, and the shock is administered without removing the electrodes from the chest wall. With most models it is possible to perform all these procedures by controls incorporated in the electrode handles. Considerable skill and training is

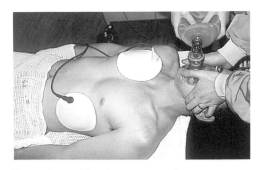

Electrode position for automated external defibrillation.

Ventricular fibrillation

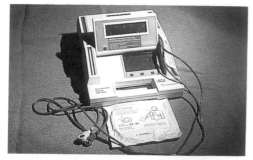

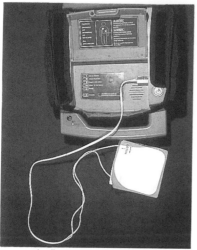

Semiautomatic advisory defibrillator.

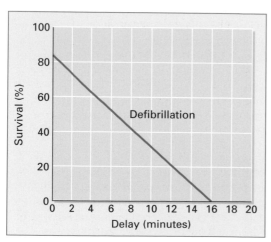

"First responder" automated defibrillators are now available in the United Kingdom. Simplicity of operation enables the device to be used by a wide range of staff. Successful use by first aiders has been reported, and the units are cheaper than many available.

necessary, mainly because of the need for interpretation of the electrocardiogram.

Semiautomatic advisory defibrillators (automated external defibrillators)

The practice of defibrillation has been revolutionised since the advent of this type of defibrillator. With the semiautomatic advisory defibrillator the tasks of interpreting the electrocardiogram and preparing for defibrillation are automated. All that is required of the operator is to recognise that cardiac arrest may have occurred and attach two large adhesive electrodes to the casualty's chest; these serve both for electrocardiographic monitoring and as defibrillator electrodes for the administration of the countershock. Instructions to the operator are provided automatically on a liquid crystal screen, and some models also incorporate a synthesised voice to re-enforce these directions. While the machine is interpreting the electrocardiogram (which takes about 10 seconds with most models currently available) the patient must be as still as possible, which means that basic life support must be interrupted. If ventricular fibrillation (or certain types of ventricular tachycardia) is recognised by the machine it will charge itself to a predetermined level and indicate to the operator when to give the shock. A pass card or manual override facility is usually incorporated which allows the machine to be used in the same way as a manual defibrillator if required. These machines offer a high degree of specificity in the recognition of ventricular fibrillation.

The advent of the semiautomatic defibrillator has brought the practice of defibrillation within the scope of a much wider range of staff than was previously possible. Training may be achieved much more rapidly and cheaply. This has enabled the ambulance service throughout the United Kingdom to equip every front line vehicle with a defibrillator. Clinical trials have shown that patients tend to receive a shock sooner when an automated rather than a manual defibrillator is used. Several groups of non-medical staff, including the police and first aid workers, have been taught to use these machines successfully.

Procedure for defibrillation

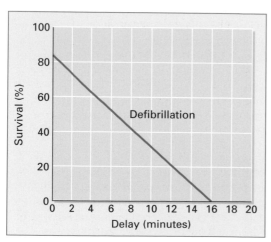

Effect of time on the success of defibrillation.

The earlier defibrillation is performed the greater the chances of success.

Guidelines for defibrillation have recently been revised by the European Resuscitation Council and endorsed by the Resuscitation Council (UK); the procedures described here are in accordance with these recommendations.

Underlying the new guidelines is the necessity to reduce to a minimum the delay in administration of defibrillatory shocks. The place of chest compression in advanced life support has been modified to allow greater opportunity for early electrical defibrillation. Although defibrillation may be possible for several minutes after cardiac arrest has occurred, the chances of success and of a favourable long term outcome are optimal for as little as 90 seconds after the onset of ventricular fibrillation; they decline thereafter with the biochemical changes that accompany circulatory and respiratory arrest. Basic life support will not reverse these changes and at best can be expected only to slow further deterioration. This concept is supported by the clinical observation that defibrillation becomes more difficult with time despite effective basic life support and by the experimental observation that the myocardial pH continues to fall during chest compression. Lack of cerebral blood flow is always a matter for concern and produces a conflict of priorities: the need for prompt defibrillatory shocks against the need for continuing basic life support to provide some cerebral circulation. On balance, the overriding initial consideration is the restoration of effective spontaneous cardiac output which provides the only means of reversing the metabolic results of circulatory arrest, and this must be achieved as rapidly as possible.

The algorithm recommended for the management of ventricular fibrillation (and pulseless ventricular tachycardia, which has the same implication for treatment) may be used for both manual and automated defibrillators.

Algorithm for treatment of ventricular fibrillation or pulseless tachycardia

In most cases of cardiac arrest basic life support will have been initiated before the algorithm is commenced. If circumstances are such that immediate defibrillation is possible, only a precordial thump should be given before definitive electrical treatment. If the first three shocks (at 200J, 200J, and 360J) can be delivered very quickly (within 30–45 seconds) then the sequence should not be interrupted by basic life support.

If the time taken to charge the defibrillator or confirm that the rhythm is still ventricular fibrillation is unduly prolonged (because old equipment is in use or because of inexperience) one or two sequences of basic life support (five chest compressions to one ventilating breath) should be administered between shocks.

The energy levels used for the first three shocks are conventional. Initial shocks at higher energy levels have not been shown to be more effective and risk greater myocardial damage. A repeated shock at 200J may succeed when an initial shock at this level has been unsuccessful because success depends on many variables that change from moment to moment. In particular the transthoracic impedence is lowered by the first shock and conditions are therefore more favourable for the second.

If three shocks are unsuccessful the prospects for recovery are reduced. The priority must now change to the provision of basic life support to preserve cerebral function and to delay as far as possible further myocardial deterioration. At this point a brief attempt should be made to intubate the patient and gain intravenous access (if this has not already been achieved). In the hospital setting these procedures may be attempted by two separate members of the resuscitation team simultaneously. Neither procedure should be allowed to cause undue delay in the continuation of basic life support or the administration of further shocks. A limited time, perhaps not more than 15 seconds, should be allowed to complete these procedures. Basic life support should be continued with 10 sequences of five compressions to one breath while preparations are made for a second set of three shocks, all at 360J. Adrenaline should be administered before these shocks if intravenous or endotracheal access is available, but the administration of the drug should not be allowed to delay attempts at defibrillation. The purpose of adrenaline is to increase the efficiency of basic life support and not to act as an adjunct to defibrillation.

After the second series of three shocks the "loop" is repeated. If intubation or intravenous access has not already been achieved each loop presents an opportunity for another attempt but always without delaying basic life support or the delivery of shocks. During each loop 1 mg of adrenaline should be given intravenously; this implies a dose of up to 1 mg every 2 minutes if shocks are given without delay. This is not considered excessive in view of the high concentration of catacholamines already present during cardiac arrest.

It is recognised that drugs given intravenously may take several minutes to exert an optimal effect, but nothing is gained by deferring further shocks as defibrillation remains the only intervention capable of restoring a spontaneous circulation. If intravenous access cannot be gained but the patient is intubated, 2 mg of adrenaline may be given by the endotracheal route. Absorption of the drug via this route, however, is much less reliable in the presence of circulatory arrest and the intravenous route remains the method of choice.

After three loops other drugs may be used if it is considered appropriate. An alkalising agent (such as sodium bicarbonate up to 50 mmol) should be given, ideally according to results of blood gas analysis. Antiarrhythmic agents may also be given after three loops, and lignocaine, bretylium, and amiodarone have all been advocated as treatment for this now desperate situation. The algorithm is not intended specifically to deny the use of agents such as calcium, magnesium, or potassium salts, whether for the treatment of known deficiences in a particular patient or on an empirical basis. No evidence exists at present in favour of these agents, and calcium has been implicated in ischaemic tissue injury.

The number of loops followed in an individual attempt at resuscitation is a matter of judgment of the clinical state and the prospects for a successful outcome. Resuscitation that was started

Ventricular fibrillation

Pulseless ventricular tachycardia

↓

Precordial thump

↓

DC shock 200 J (1)

↓

DC shock 200 J (2)

↓

DC shock 360 J (3)

↓

If not done already:
- intubate
- establish intravenous
- access

↓

Adrenaline 1 mg intravenously

↓

10 Sequences of 5:1 compression/ventilation

↓

DC shock 360 J (4)

↓

DC shock 360 J (5)

↓

DC shock 360 J (6)

Notes:

(1) The interval between shocks 3 and 4 should not exceed 2 minutes

(2) Adrenaline should be given during each loop – ie, every 2 to 3 minutes

(3) Continue loops for as long as defibrillation is indicated

(4) After 3 loops consider:
- an alkalising agent
- an antiarrhythmic agent

Algorithm for managing ventricular fibrillation or pulseless ventricular tachycardia.

appropriately should not usually be abandoned while the rhythm is still recognisable ventricular fibrillation, whereas the development of persistent asystole is an indication that the prospects of success are slim. Few situations would call for efforts continuing for more than one hour, although cardiac arrest in children and in the presence of hypothermia or drug overdose should always be considered on their merits. Before attempts at defibrillation are abandoned the possibility of a change of electrode position or even a change of defibrillator should be considered.

Safety

Care is needed to ensure that the use of a defibrillator is not accompanied by any risk to staff participating in the resuscitation attempt. When defibrillation is carried out it is essential that no part of any member of the team is in direct contact with the casualty. The operator must shout "stand clear" and check that all those present have done so before giving the shock. There are traps for the unwary: wet surroundings or clothing are dangerous; intravenous infusion equipment must not be held by helpers; the operator must be certain not to touch any part of the electrode surface; and care is needed to ensure that excess electrode gel does not allow an electrical arc across the surface of the chest wall. Similarly, care is needed to ensure that electrode gel does not spread from the chest wall to the operator's hands; the use of gel impregnated pads reduces this risk.

Further reading

Advanced Life Support Working Party of the European Resuscitation Council. Guidelines for advanced life support. *Resuscitation* 1992; **24**: 111–22.

von Planta M, Chamberlain DA. Drug treatment of arrhythmias during cardiopulmonary resuscitation. A statement for the Advanced Life Support Working Party of the European Resuscitation Council. *Resuscitation* 1992; **24**: 227–32.

Waller DG. Treatment and prevention of ventricular defibrillation: are there better agents? *Resuscitation* 1991; **22**: 159–66.

Robertson C. Pre-cordial thump and cough techniques in advanced life support. *Resuscitation* 1992; **24**: 133–5.

Bossaerts L. Koster R. Defibrillation methods and strategies. *Resuscitation* 1992; **24**: 211–25.

Cummins RO. From concept to standard of care? Review of the clinical experience with automated external defibrillators. *Ann Emerg Med* 1989; **18**: 1269–76.

3 ASYSTOLE AND ELECTROMECHANICAL DISSOCIATION

Michael Colquhoun, A John Camm

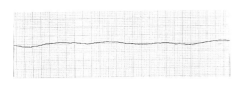

Asystole: baseline drift is present. The ECG is rarely a completely straight line in asystole.

Asystole

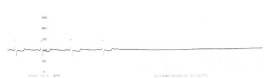

The onset of asystole complicating complete heart block.

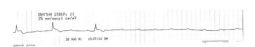

Onset of asystole due to sino-atrial block.

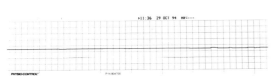

If the ECG appears as a straight line the leads, gain, and electrical connections must be checked.

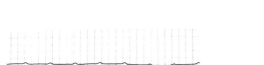

Ventricular asystole. Persistent P waves due to atrial depolarisation are seen.

There are three main mechanisms of cardiac arrest: ventricular fibrillation, ventricular asystole, and electromechanical dissociation. Outside hospital most cases of cardiac arrest (80–90%) are due to ventricular fibrillation, which is often preceded by ventricular tachycardia; asystole accounts for about 10% and electromechanical dissociation for less than 5%. The situation is different in hospital, where about 25% of cardiac arrests are due to asystole and electromechanical dissociation is not uncommon. Cardiac arrest due either to asystole or electromechanical dissociation is more difficult to treat than ventricular fibrillation and carries a much worse prognosis.

In asystolic cardiac arrest ventricular standstill is present because of the suppression of all natural or artificial cardiac pacemakers. Under normal circumstances an idioventricular rhythm will maintain cardiac output when either the supraventricular pacemakers fail or atrioventricular conduction is interrupted. Myocardial disease, electrolyte disturbance, anoxia, or drugs may suppress this rhythm and cause asystole. Excessive cholinergic activity may suddenly depress sinus or atrioventricular node function and cause asystole, especially when sympathetic tone is reduced, for example by ischaemia, infarction, or β blockade.

Electrocardiographic appearance

Asystole is diagnosed when no ventricular activity can be seen on the electrocardiogram. Atrial and ventricular asystole usually coexist so that the electrocardiogram is a straight line with no recognisable deflections. This line will, however, be distorted by base line drift, electrical interference, respiratory movements, and cardiopulmonary resuscitation. A completely straight line usually means that a monitoring lead has become disconnected. Ventricular fibrillation may be mistaken for asystole if one lead only is monitored or the fibrillatory activity is of low amplitude. Because ventricular fibrillation is so readily treatable and resuscitation is therefore more likely to be successful, it is vital that great care is taken before diagnosing asystole. The electrocardiograph leads, connections, gain, and brilliance of the monitor must be checked. All contact with the patient should cease briefly to reduce the possibility of interference. An alternative ECG lead should be recorded when the monitor has this facility or the defibrillator electrodes moved to different positions.

On occasions atrial activity may continue for a short time after the onset of ventricular asystole. The electrocardiogram in this case will show a straight line interrupted by P waves but with no evidence of ventricular depolarisation.

Management

Careful thought should be given before undertaking prolonged attempts at resuscitation in asystolic cardiac arrest. If there is any possibility that the rhythm could be fine ventricular fibrillation, initial treatment should follow the algorithm for ventricular fibrillation (chapter 2). Little harm will result from this approach, and the delay in the implementation of the asystole algorithm should be slight. It is important to remember than an automated defibrillator may not recognise fine ventricular fibrillation when the amplitude of the fibrillatory waves is below the sensitivity of the instrument. Under these circumstances the machine will determine that a shock is inappropriate and time will be wasted. It is then necessary to convert the machine to the manual mode of operation before defibrillation can be carried out.

The initial sequence of defibrillation, if used, should be followed by tracheal intubation, the securing of intravenous access, and the administration of drugs. Adrenaline is given to enhance the effectiveness of basic life support through the peripheral vasoconstriction produced by its α adrenergic effect. In addition the β adrenergic effect may increase the rate of discharge of the sinoatrial node and may facilitate the production of an idioventricular rhythm. Atropine is given in a dose that blocks vagal tone completely under normal circumstances (3 mg), and only a single dose is required. This will relieve cholinergic depression of sinus and atrioventricular node function.

There is no convincing evidence from either animal work or clinical trials that atropine is useful in asystolic cardiac arrest. Asystole carries a grave prognosis, however, and there are anecdotal reports of success after the administration of atropine; moreover it is unlikely to be harmful in this situation.

Undue delay or interruption in the sequence of basic life support (for example, when performing intubation or inserting intravenous lines) must be avoided. In the absence of recognisable electrical activity further loops of the algorithm should be considered. These consist of the injection of 1 mg of adrenaline and 10 cycles of basic life support. If no response has been obtained after three such loops the use of high dose adrenaline (5 mg) should be considered, though its value, like that of atropine, is unproved.

Cardiac pacing is often effective when applied to patients with asystole due to atrioventricular block or failure of sinus node discharge. It is less likely to be successful when asystole follows extensive myocardial impairment or systemic metabolic upset. It should be considered if any electrical activity is evident, particularly when there are P waves without ventricular complexes or if a very slow ventricular rhythm is present.

Transvenous pacing is the method of choice if the equipment and skills are available. Non-invasive transthoracic pacing may buy time until this can be established and has proved successful for the emergency treatment of bradycardia; results are usually disappointing in asystolic cardiac arrest. It does, however, avoid the trauma of transcutaneous pacing (through a needle inserted directly into the myocardium) and the technical difficulties of oesophageal pacing (see chapter 20).

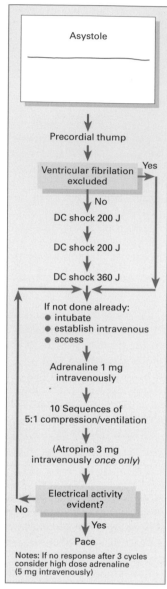

Algorithm for managing asystole.

Hypoxia

Profound hypoxia that can occur for example, in severe asthma, may give rise to asystole. Patients must be intubated and ventilated with 100% oxygen; prolonged attempts at resuscitation are always indicated in this setting and may be successful as they may be in the presence of hypothermia.

Electromechanical dissociation

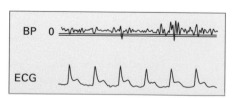

Electromechanical dissociation in a patient with acute myocardial infarction. Despite an apparently near normal cardiac rhythm there was no blood pressure.

The term electromechanical dissociation signifies the features of cardiac arrest despite normal (or near normal) electrical excitation. The diagnosis is made from a combination of the clinical absence of cardiac output with the presence of a rhythm on the monitor that would normally be accompanied by good ventricular function.

The causes can be divided into two broad categories. In primary electromechanical dissociation there is failure of the excitation contraction coupling process that results in profound loss of cardiac output. Causes include massive myocardial infarction (particularly inferior wall), poisoning with drugs (β blockers, calcium antagonists) or toxins, and electrolyte disturbance (hypocalcaemia; hyperkalaemia). In secondary electromechanical dissociation mechanical barriers to

Causes of electromechanical dissociation

1 *Primary electromechanical dissociation (failure of excitation-contraction coupling)*
- Myocardial infarction (particularly inferior wall)
- Drugs (β blockers and calcium antagonists) or toxins
- Electrolyte abnormalities (such as hypocalcaemia, hyperkalaemia)
- Atrial thrombus or tumour (myxoma)

2 *Secondary electromechanical dissociation (mechanical embarrassment to cardiac output)*
- Tension pneumothorax
- Pericardial tamponade
- Cardiac rupture
- Pulmonary embolism
- Prosthetic heart valve occlusion
- Hypovolaemia

ventricular filling or cardiac output are present. Causes include tension pneumothorax, pericardial tamponade, cardiac rupture, pulmonary embolism, occlusion of prosthetic heart valve, and hypovolaemia. Treatment in all cases is directed towards the underlying cause.

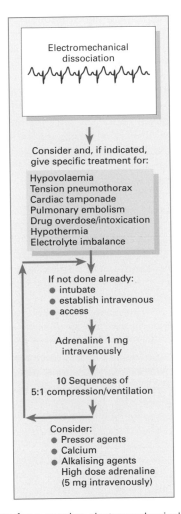

Algorithm for managing electromechanical dissociation.

The search for and recognition of specific correctable causes of electromechanical dissociation is of paramount importance; the principal ones are listed in the algorithm.

If there is no evidence of a specific cause cardiopulmonary resuscitation should be continued with the usual sequence of tracheal intubation, establishment of venous access, and administration of adrenaline as described in the algorithm. There is no evidence that the routine use of pressor agents, calcium chloride, alkalising agents, or high dose adrenaline is beneficial, although in specific circumstances one or more of these may be of value. Calcium (as intravenous calcium chloride) is specifically indicated when hypocalcaemia, hyperkalaemia, or calcium antagonist toxicity is present. Hypercalcaemia and calcium overload, sufficient to cause cardiac or cerebral cell death, however, may complicate its use.

Further reading

Guidelines for advanced life support. A statement by the Advanced Life Support Working Party of the European Resuscitation Council, 1992. *Resuscitation* 1992; **24**: 111–21.

Evans TR, Morgensen L. Pharmacological treatment of asystole and electromechanical dissociation. *Resuscitation* 1991; **22**: 167–72.

Cripps T, Camm AJ. The management of electromechanical dissociation. *Resuscitation* 1991; **22**: 173–80.

4 MANAGEMENT OF THE PERI-ARREST ARRHYTHMIAS

Michael Colquhoun, T R Evans, Douglas Chamberlain, Richard Vincent

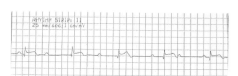

Complete heart block complicating inferior infarction: narrow QRS complex.

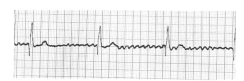

Atrial fibrillation with complete heart block. Bradycardia may arise for many reasons. Assessment of the cardiac output is essential.

Asystole lasting several seconds due to sino-atrial block.

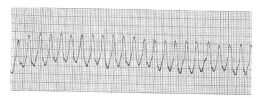

Rapid broad complex tachycardia: if the patient is unconscious, without a pulse, treatment is the same as ventricular fibrillation.

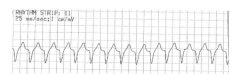

Broad complex tachycardia: treatment will depend on the presence of adverse signs.

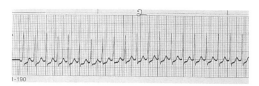

Narrow complex tachycardia.

In chapters 2 and 3 the treatment of the arrhythmias that most commonly cause cardiac arrest has been described. Their management follows the guidelines produced by the European Resuscitation Council for the management of ventricular fibrillation, pulseless ventricular tachycardia, asystole, and electromechanical dissociation.

A coordinated strategy to reduce death from cardiac arrest must also include measures to prevent and treat other potentially lethal arrhythmias that may precede cardiac arrest or complicate the early period after resuscitation. Ventricular fibrillation, for example, is often triggered by another arrhythmia; this may recur after successful defibrillation or a different arrhythmia may develop. Either factor will compromise the patient's chance of survival. The first members of staff with advanced skills in cardiac life support who manage patients with cardiac arrest are not usually skilled in the management of complex arrhythmias; these guidelines are designed to help those without extensive training who manage most cases.

The European Resuscitation Council has recently published guidelines for the initial management of peri-arrest arrhythmias,[1] and this chapter is based on these guidelines, which complement others in chapters 2 and 3. The intention is that they should be straightforward in their application and, as far as possible, be applicable in all European countries notwithstanding different traditions of antiarrhythmic treatment. An important component of the recommendations is guidance on when expert help might reasonably be requested.

The guidelines are summarised in three algorithms: the first for bradycardia and intracardiac conduction block, the second for the management of broad complex tachycardia, and the third for the management of narrow complex tachycardia. In the circumstances under discussion broad complex tachycardia will almost always be due to ventricular tachycardia; the alternative diagnosis (supraventricular tachycardia conducted with aberration) can, from a practical point of view, be disregarded. This applies particularly to patients with ischaemic heart disease, which remains the commonest cause of cardiac arrest in adults.

Three important reservations regarding the application of the algorithms must be emphasised at the outset. Firstly, it is impossible to encompass all eventualities that could possibly occur; a situation may well arise that calls for measures different from those suggested. Secondly, the advice to obtain expert help assumes that the practitioner in charge does not have the skill necessary for the definitive management of the arrhythmia. Such skills might, however, be possessed by practitioners in any one of several disciplines and are by no means confined to cardiologists. Thirdly, the special situation that exists in relation to arrhythmias complicating poisoning and drug overdose is not included; expert help is manadatory.

Two hazards of treatment must be mentioned. In the first place, all antiarrhythmic strategies (whether physical manoeuvres, pharmacological agents, or electrical treatments) may also cause arrhythmias—that is, they may they themselves be pro-arrhythmic. Thus, deterioration in the patient's condition may occur as a result of treatment rather than because of a lack of effect. In the second place antiarrhythmic drugs, particularly when used in high dosage or in combination, may cause myocardial depression and hypotension. The hazards of treatment may therefore include deterioration in cardiac rhythm and in force of contraction; decisions on the management of individual patients must be made carefully, especially in refractory cases.

The three algorithms shown are produced by the European Resuscitation Council. It is implicit in all three that oxygen is usually appropriate in a setting that threatens or follows cardiac arrest.

Bradycardia and conduction block

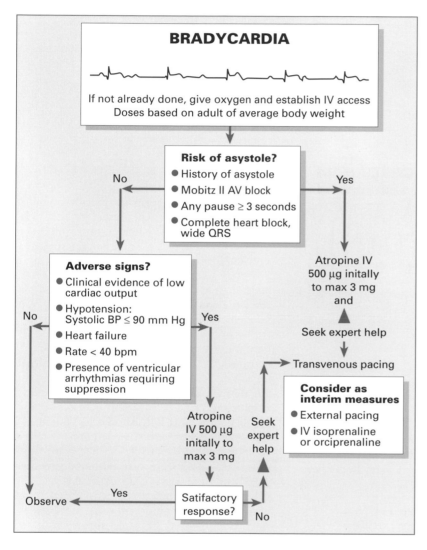

BRADYCARDIA

If not already done, give oxygen and establish IV access
Doses based on adult of average body weight

Risk of asystole?
● History of asystole
● Mobitz II AV block
● Any pause ≥ 3 seconds
● Complete heart block, wide QRS

No — Yes

Adverse signs?
● Clinical evidence of low cardiac output
● Hypotension: Systolic BP ≤ 90 mm Hg
● Heart failure
● Rate < 40 bpm
● Presence of ventricular arrhythmias requiring suppression

No — Yes

Atropine IV 500 µg initally to max 3 mg

Seek expert help

Satifactory response?

Yes — Observe

No

Atropine IV 500 µg initially to max 3 mg and

Seek expert help

Transvenous pacing

Consider as interim measures
● External pacing
● IV isoprenaline or orciprenaline

Bradycardia is defined as a ventricular rate below 60 beats/min. Such absolute bradycardia is easily recognised, but in the circumstances under discussion it is also important to recognise the patient whose heart rate may be greater than 60 beats/min yet be inappropriately slow for his or her haemodynamic state; that is a relative bradycardia.

The treatment of bradycardia and conduction block depends on whether there is an appreciable risk of asystole supervening. Four settings are recognised as of paramount importance: a previous episode of asystole, Mobitz type II atrioventricular block, a pause equal to or greater than 3 seconds (regardless of cause), and the presence of complete heart block with a wide QRS complex. Third degree (complete) atrioventricular block with a narrow QRS complex is not in itself an indication for treatment because the atrioventricular junctional pacemaker present in these circumstances often provides an adequate, stable, ventricular rate.

If there is thought to be a definite risk of asystole, intravenous access should be established and atropine administered while arrangements are made for transvenous pacing. In many cases expert help will be required for this, and if the patient's condition is critical and the necessary equipment is available external pacing (after sedation if necessary) should be used. Judicious use of isoprenaline is an alternative strategy. A starting dose of 1 µg a minute is usually used; 2·5 mg isoprenaline dissolved in 500 ml of carrier solution and administered through an infusion pump at 0·2 ml a minute will provide this infusion rate. The dose may be increased rapidly, but regard should be paid to the risk of precipitating or aggravating ventricular arrhythmias. Isoprenaline increases myocardial consumption of oxygen and may cause serious reduction in plasma potassium concentrations.

If there is no perceived risk of the occurrence of asystole the presence or absence of adverse clinical signs should be noted. These include clinical evidence of a low cardiac output because of impaired myocardial function, a very low absolute heart rate (less than 40 beats/min), and the emergence of ventricular tachyarrhythmias that require suppression. If such signs are absent then continued observation and monitoring of the patient are required. If one or more adverse signs are present, atropine should be administered in an initial dose of 500 or 600 µg by slow intravenous injection. Incremental doses to a maximum total dose of 3 mg may be given at intervals of a few minutes; a total dose higher than 3 mg will produce no additional benefit but will increase the severity of unwanted effects. A satisfactory response to atropine will indicate the need for continued observation; failure to respond indicates the need for transvenous pacing.

The interim measures already described may be appropriate if there

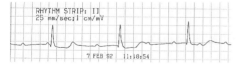

Complete heart block: wide QRS duration ≥ 100 milliseconds.

is likely to be appreciable delay before cardiac pacing can be established. When the successful effect of atropine is shortlived or large doses have to be repeated, transvenous pacing will usually be required for long-lasting stabilisation.

Broad complex tachycardia

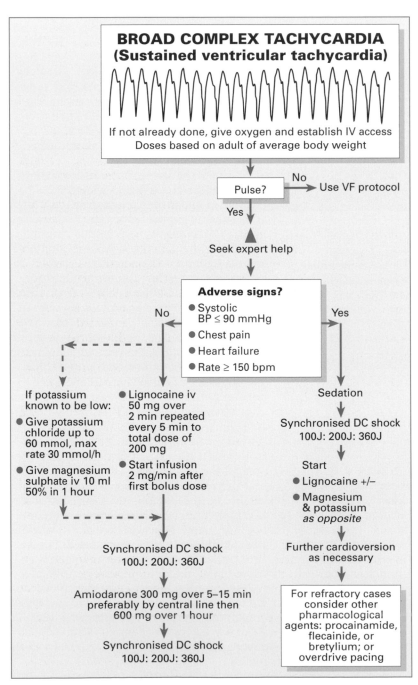

In the context of resuscitation, broad complex tachycardia will almost invariably be ventricular in origin. Little harm results if supraventricular tachycardia is treated as a ventricular arrhythmia, whereas the converse error may have serious consequences. The first question that determines management is whether or not there is a palpable pulse. With pulseless ventricular tachycardia the patient will be unconscious and should be treated in the same way as for ventricular fibrillation according to the guidelines already described in chapter 2.

If there is a palpable pulse oxygen should be administered and intravenous access established; expert help should be sought at this stage. If there are adverse clinical signs (the presence of ischaemic cardiac pain, signs of heart failure with a systolic blood pressure of 90 mmHg or less, or a ventricular rate of 150 beats/min or more) the arrhythmia should be regarded as an emergency. In most cases synchronised direct current cardioversion should be considered after appropriate sedation. In refractory cases if the plasma potassium concentration is known to be less than 3·6 mmol/l (especially in the context of recent myocardial infarction) most authorities recommend an infusion of potassium and magnesium while further attempts at cardioversion are prepared. If this is unsuccessful or the arrhythmia recurs lignocaine should be administered. If the arrhythmia still remains refractory an alternative agent such as flecainide, propafenone, bretylium, or procainamide may be successful. When the necessary skill is available overdrive pacing may also be considered.

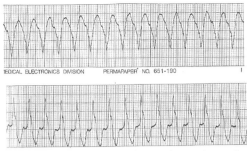

The morphology of broad complex tachycardia may present different forms: Leads V₁ (upper trace) and V₆ (lower trace) recorded in the same patient.

In the absence of adverse signs lignocaine may be given in conventional doses. If the potassium concentration is known to be low (if it is not known it must be measured as a matter of urgency) an infusion of potassium and magnesium is recommended to help prevent recurrent rhythm disturbances. If lignocaine is ineffective, synchronised direct current cardioversion should be considered as the next stage in treatment. When the arrhythmia remains refractory and there are no adverse signs amiodarone should be given by slow intravenous injection (300 mg over 5–15 minutes preferably through a central line) and followed by an intravenous infusion of a further 600 mg over one hour. If this is ineffective, further attempts at synchronised cardioversion should be made after an hour has elapsed for the drug to produce its powerful antiarrhythmic effects. Should the patient's condition deteriorate and adverse signs develop immediate electrical cardioversion should be undertaken.

Narrow complex tachycardia

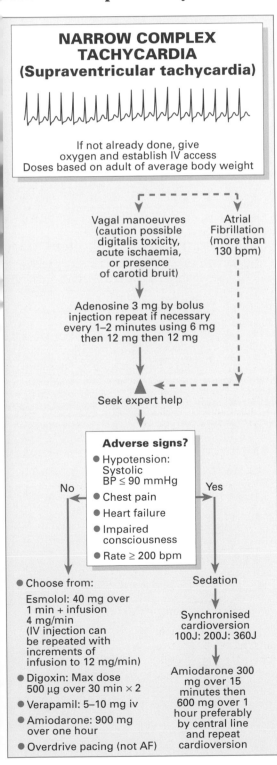

Narrow complex tachycardia will virtually always be supraventricular in origin – that is, the tachycardia passes through the atrioventricular node. Supraventricular tachycardias are usually less dangerous than those of ventricular origin and only rarely occur after successful treatment of ventricular tachyarrhythmias, although they are a recognised trigger for the development of ventricular fibrillation in vulnerable patients. Atrial fibrillation, on the other hand, occurs commonly in the early period after resuscitation.

As in the treatment of other arrhythmias in life threatening situations oxygen should be given and intravenous access should be secured as soon as possible. Vagotonic manoeuvres (particularly the Valsava manoeuvre or carotid sinus massage) should always be considered in the management of supraventricular tachycardia but are not always advisable. In the context of resuscitation there are hazards that require emphasis; profound vagotonic tone may cause sudden bradycardia and trigger ventricular fibrillation, particularly in the presence of acute ischaemia or digitalis toxicity. Carotid sinus massage may produce rupture of an atheromatous plaque which may lead to cerebral embolism.

The drug of choice for the treatment of a regular supraventricular tachycardia is adenosine, which should be given by rapid intravenous injection as it is rapidly eliminated from the circulation. An initial dose of 3 mg is recommended, although this will be effective in only a few cases. Incremental doses can be given every one to two minutes with up to two injections of 12 mg if necessary. If adenosine is unsuccessful at terminating supraventricular tachycardia or if atrial fibrillation at a ventricular rate of more than 130 beats/min is present expert help should be sought. At this point management will depend on whether adverse signs (cardiac failure, hypotension, ischaemic cardiac pain, impaired consciousness, or a rate equal to or greater than 200 beats/min) are present. In the presence of one or more adverse factors treatment should consist of synchronised direct current cardioversion after appropriate sedation. If this is unsuccessful it should be repeated after an intravenous injection and subsequent infusion of amiodarone using the same regimen described earlier for the treatment of broad complex tachycardia. If there is no perceived urgency, then up to an hour may elapse before further attempts at cardioversion are made. Circumstances, however, may dictate a shorter time interval.

Management of the peri-arrest arrhythmias

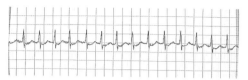

Narrow complex tachycardia.

In the absence of adverse signs intravenous amiodarone is an alternative initial treatment, as is overdrive pacing when the skill is available. Other intravenous drug treatments that may be considered are esmolol (a short acting β blocker), digoxin, or verapamil. Caution is necessary with verapamil. Although this drug is widely used and is very often successful in supraventricular tachycardia, there are circumstances in which it is hazardous. These include arrhythmias associated with Wolff-Parkinson-White syndrome, tachycardias that are ventricular in origin, and in some of the supraventricular arrhythmias of childhood. The potential serious interaction between verapamil and β adrenergic blocking agents must also be considered, particularly when both drugs have been administered intravenously.

We acknowledge use of the European Resuscitation Council guidelines and algorithms for the treatment of peri-arrest arrhythmias on which the recommendations in this chapter are based.

1. Peri-arrest arrhythmias (Management of arrhythmias associated with cardiac arrest). A statement by the Advanced Life Support Committee of the European Resuscitation Council, 1994; **28**: 151–9

5 THE AIRWAY AT RISK

R S Simons

Failure to maintain a patent airway is a well recognised cause of avoidable death in unconscious patients. The principles of airway management during cardiac arrest or after major trauma are the same as those during anaesthesia.

Airway patency

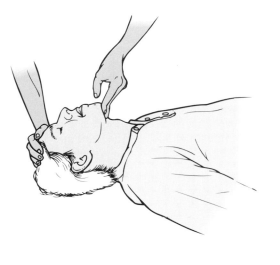

Airway patency may be impaired by the loss of normal muscle tone or by obstruction. This includes contamination by foreign material from the mouth, nasopharynx, oesophagus, or stomach.

In the unconscious patient relaxation of the tongue, neck, and pharyngeal muscles causes soft tissue obstruction of the supraglottic airway. This may be corrected by the techniques of head tilt with jaw lift or jaw thrust. The use of head tilt will relieve obstruction in 80% of patients but should not be used if a cervical spine injury is suspected. Chin lift or jaw thrust will further improve airway patency but will tend to oppose the lips. With practice, chin lift and jaw thrust can be performed without causing cervical spine movement. In some patients, airway obstruction may be particularly noticeable during expiration, due to the flap-valve effect of the soft palate against the nasopharyngeal tissues, as occurs in snoring.

Recovery posture

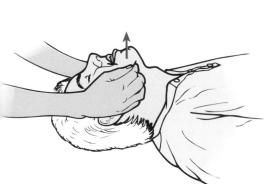

Patients with adequate spontaneous ventilation and circulation who cannot safeguard their own airway will be at risk of developing airway obstruction in the supine position. Turning the patient laterally into the coma or recovery position allows the tongue to fall forward, with less risk of pharyngeal obstruction; fluid in the mouth can then drain outwards instead of soiling the trachea and lungs.

Recovery positions range from a true lateral posture (with either upper or lower leg flexed) to the semiprone posture, depending on the relative tilt of the pelvis and shoulders and the attitude of the arms. The subject may lie on either side. Emergency tracheal intubation may arguably be performed more easily with the patient lying on the left side, but a full stomach is more liable to be compressed and cause regurgitation in this position. The semiprone posture provides better drainage from the mouth and greater stability during transport, but the casualty's face, colour, and chest movement are more difficult to observe; ventilation may also be impaired. Moreover, the patient is inconveniently positioned if he or she needs to be returned to the supine position for further resuscitation manoeuvres.

Spinal injury

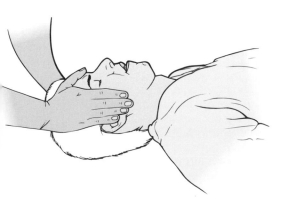

The casualty with suspected spinal injuries requires careful handling and should be managed in the supine aligned position, with constant attention to the airway. The semiprone recovery position should not be used because considerable rotation of the neck is required to prevent the patient lying face downwards. If the patient must be turned, he or she should be "log rolled" into a true lateral position by several rescuers in unison, taking care to avoid rotation or flexion of the spine, especially the cervical spine.

If the head or upper chest is injured, bony neck injury should be assumed to be present until excluded by lateral cervical spine radiography and examination by a specialist. The head and neck should be maintained in a neutral position by using in line manual immobilisation, a semirigid collar, sandbags, a spinal board, and securing straps. The neck must not be actively flexed or extended during chin lift, jaw thrust, or when inserting airway adjuncts. If tracheal intubation is required in the spontaneously breathing patient, blind nasal or fibre optic intubation may be preferred.

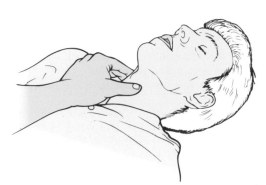

Sellick's manoeuvre of cricoid pressure.

Vomiting and regurgitation

Rescuers should always be aware of the risk of contamination of the unprotected airway by fluid or solid debris.

Vomiting and regurgitation are subtly different. Vomiting is an active process of stomach contraction with retrograde propulsion up the oesophagus. It occurs more commonly during lighter levels of unconsciousness or when cerebral perfusion improves after resuscitation from cardiac arrest. Prodromal retching may allow time to place the patient in the lateral recovery position or head down (Trendelenburg) tilt, and prepare for suction or manual removal of debris from the mouth and pharynx.

Regurgitation is a passive and often silent flow of stomach contents (typically fluid) retrogradely up the oesophagus, with the risk of inhalation and soiling of the lungs; acidic gastric fluid may cause severe chemical pneumonitis. Failure to maintain a clear airway during spontaneous ventilation may encourage regurgitation because the negative intrathoracic pressure developed during obstructed inspiration may encourage aspiration of gastric contents across a weak mucosal flap valve between the stomach and oesophagus. Recent food or fluid ingestion, obesity, hiatus hernia, intestinal obstruction, and late pregnancy all make regurgitation more likely to occur during resuscitation. Chest compression over the lower sternum increases the risk of regurgitation as well as risking damage to abdominal organs.

Gaseous distention of the stomach increases the likelihood of regurgitation, and restricts chest expansion. Inadvertent gastric distension may occur during artificial ventilation, especially if the lungs are inflated rapidly with large tidal volumes and high inflation pressures. This is particularly likely to happen when gas powered resuscitators are employed in conjunction with facemasks. These resuscitators should therefore be used only when the trachea has been intubated.

The cricoid pressure manoeuvre, recommended by Sellick,[1] is well known to anaesthetists. Compression of the oesophagus between the cricoid ring and the sixth cervical vertebra prevents passive regurgitation, but should not be applied during active vomiting. The manoeuvre also helps to prevent gastric inflation during cardiopulmonary resuscitation but requires the presence of another rescuer.

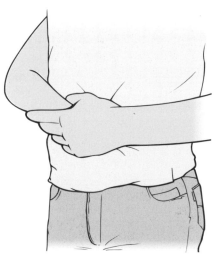

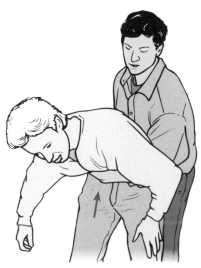

Heimlich's abdominal thrust.

Choking

Asphyxia due to impaction of food or other foreign body in the upper airway is a dramatic and frightening event. In the conscious patient, back blows and abdominal thrusts (the Heimlich manoeuvre) have been widely recommended. Attempts may be made to provoke coughing or vomiting. If respiratory obstruction persists the patient will become unconscious and collapse. The supine casualty may be given further abdominal thrusts, and manual attempts at pharyngeal disimpaction should be undertaken. Visual inspection of the throat with a laryngoscope and the use of Magill forceps or suction is desirable, but such equipment is seldom available at the time of need.

If attempts at relieving choking are unsuccessful, the final hypoxic arrest may be indistinguishable from other types of cardiac arrest. Treatment should follow the ABC (airway, breathing, and circulation) routine, although ventilation may be difficult or impossible to perform. The act of forceful chest compression may, however, clear the offending object from the laryngopharynx.

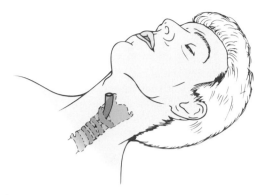

Cricothyrotomy (laryngotomy).

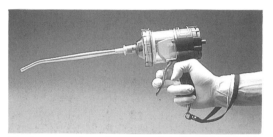

Hand operated suction pump (vitallograph).

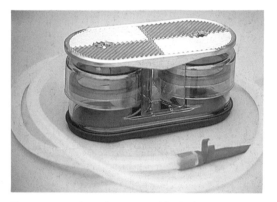

Foot operated suction pump (Ambu).

Surgical intervention

If the upper airway (above the vocal cords) remains obstructed—for example, due to a foreign body, maxillo-facial trauma, extrinsic pressure, or inflammation, cricothyrotomy (laryngotomy) may be lifesaving and should not be unduly delayed. Any strong knife, scissor point, large bore cannula, or similar instrument can be used to create an opening through the cricothyroid membrane, in the absence of surgical instruments. An opening of 5–7 mm diameter is made and needs to be maintained with an appropriate hollow tube. Artificial ventilation may be applied directly to the orifice or the tube inserted.

Jet ventilation with oxygen at 40–50 psi (3 bar) applied to a 12–14 gauge cannula cricothyrotomy can be used as an emergency measure for for up to 45 minutes pending a surgical cricothyrotomy or formal tracheostomy. It is important to maintain a 1 sec : 4 sec inflation:exhalation cycle when using this technique to allow adequate time for expiration.

Cricothyrotomy is contraindicated in children under 12 years of age. Tracheostomy is technically difficult and should be undertaken only as a formal surgical procedure under optimum conditions.

Suction

Equipment for suction clearance of the oropharynx and airways is essential for the provision of comprehensive life support. When choosing one of the many devices available, considerations of cost, portability, and power supply are paramount. Devices powered by electricity or compressed gas risk exhaustion of the power supply at a critical time; battery operated devices require regular recharging or battery replacement. Hand or foot operated pumps are particularly suitable for field use and suit the occasional user. Ease of cleaning and reassembly are other important factors. Rigid, wide bore plastic or metal suction cannulas can be supplemented by the use of soft plastic suction catheters when necessary. A suction booster which traps fluid debris in a reservoir close to the patient may improve suction capability.

Airway support and ventilation devices

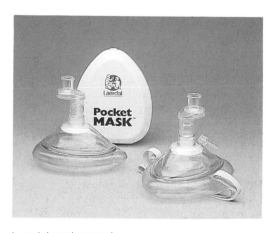

Laerdal pocket mask.

Resuscitation airways are devices which may variously be used to improve airway patency, provide a mouthpiece for artificial ventilation, or provide oxygen enrichment. Some afford protection to the rescuer and some isolate the airway against pulmonary soiling from gastric aspiration.

Because of concern about the risk of bacterial or viral infection, particularly by hepatitis or HIV, during mouth to mouth resuscitation there has been an increasing demand for small, inexpensive airway adjuncts which prevent direct patient contact.

Barrier or shield devices

Most consist of a plastic sheet with a central airway that incorporates a one-way patient valve or filter. They are compact and inexpensive, but are difficult to seal effectively; several present a high resistance to rescuer inflation, especially when wet. Most do not have a sufficiently long oral tube to maintain airway patency.

Tongue support

The classic curved oral Guedel airway used in anaesthesia improves airway patency but requires supplementary jaw support. In lightly

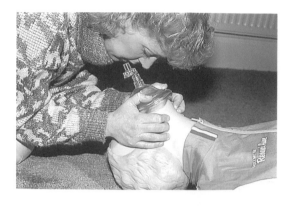

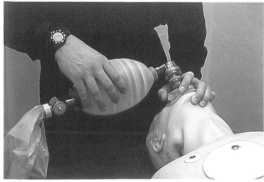

Nurses using Laerdal pocket mask. Supplemental oxygen is added to an inlet port in the mask.

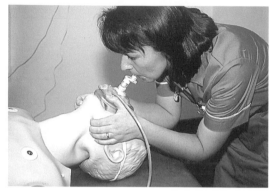

Pulse oximeter.

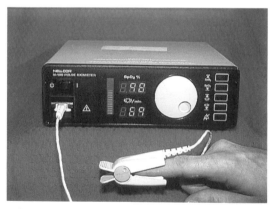

Bag-mask ventilation, one operator.

unconscious patients oropharyngeal stimulation may induce vomiting. Soft nasopharyngeal tubes are less likely to do this but may cause nasopharyngeal bleeding; they require skill to insert. These simple airways do not protrude from the face and are therefore suitable for use in combination with mask ventilation.

Several disposable airway adjuncts exist that maintain oropharyngeal patency while also providing a lip seal that acts as a port for rescuer ventilation. Apart from the Safar-S double-ended airway, most now incorporate valves or filters for rescuer protection. Examples include the Brook, Hilt, Lifeway, and Sussex airways. When assessing their suitability consideration should be given to size, weight, airway patency, mouth seal, rescuer protection, inflow resistance, and cost.

Ventilation masks

The use of ventilation masks during expired air resuscitation offers the rescuer protection against direct patient contact, especially when used in conjunction with a non-rebreathing valve or filter. The rescuer seals the mask on the casualty's face using a firm two handed grip and blows through the mask while lifting the patient's jaw. If the casualty's lips are opposed, only limited air flow may be possible, through the nose, and obstructed expiration may be unrecognised in some subjects. The insertion of oral or nasal airways is therefore advisable when using mask ventilation.

Several manufacturers produce transparent masks with well fitting air filled cuffs that provide an effective seal on the casualty's face. They may incorporate valves through which the rescuer can conduct mouth to mask ventilation. Where the valve is detachable the mask orifice should be the standard size that accommodates a self inflating bag (outside diameter 22 mm/inside diameter 15 mm), so that bag-valve-mask ventilation may be undertaken. Some rescue masks embody an inlet port for supplementary oxygen, although in an emergency an oxygen delivery tube can be introduced under the mask cuff or clenched in the rescuer's mouth. At least one manufacturer produces a pocket mask with slim-line carry case, complete with rescuer valve and oxygen inlet port.

Supplementary oxygen

Oxygen should always be used during cardiopulmonary emergencies as soon as it is available. Room air contains 21% oxygen and expired air only 16%. In shock, a low cardiac output together with ventilation-perfusion mismatch result in severe hypoxaemia. An inspired oxygen concentration of 80–100% is desirable. Oxygen is also harmless for most patients. Only a few patients with chronic obstructive lung disease and CO_2 retention (type II respiratory failure or "blue bloaters") manifest underventilation with excessive oxygen therapy, though if severely hypoxic they too require optimal oxygenation and ventilation. For spontaneously breathing or ventilated patients oxygen can be supplied either to a mask, as described above, or to an oxygen reservoir behind the ventilation bag as explained below.

An improvement in the patient's colour is a sign of improved tissue oxygenation. Portable oximeters with finger or ear probes are increasingly used to measure arterial oxygen saturation, provided an adequate pulsatile blood flow is required. Normal arterial saturation is in excess of 93% compared to a venous saturation of about 75%. Arterial oxygen saturation should be maintained above 90% by combining adequate ventilation with oxygen supplementation.

Bag-valve devices

A self refilling manual resuscitation bag can be attached to the mask to facilitate bag-valve-mask ventilation with air and supplementary oxygen at inspiratory volumes of 800–1000 ml. The technique requires additional training because it is difficult to apply the mask securely and lift the jaw with one hand, while squeezing the bag with the other. If ventilation is ineffective a two handed grip on the mask should be maintained with an additional rescuer squeezing the bag.

The addition of oxygen at a flow rate of 8–12 l/min via an oxygen reservoir will ensure preferential refilling of the resuscitation bag so as

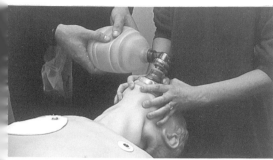

Bag-mask ventilation, two operators.

to maintain inspired oxygen levels of 80–95%. Oxygen supplementation through a side port on the mask will provide only 35–50% inspired concentration.

Studies of the different methods of ventilation indicate that for those rescuers whose daily activities do not require anaesthetic or resuscitative skills, effective ventilatory volumes are more easily achieved by mouth to mask ventilation than by mouth to mouth or bag-valve-mask ventilation.

Health care professionals should not be expected to perform unprotected mouth to mouth resuscitation and skill expectation, training, frequency of use, and cost will largely determine the equipment required.

Airway isolation

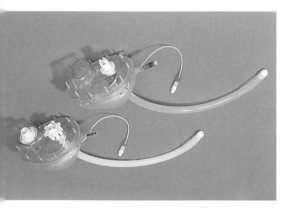

Oesophageal obturators. Esophageal Obturator Airway (upper) and Esophageal Gastric Tube Airway (lower).

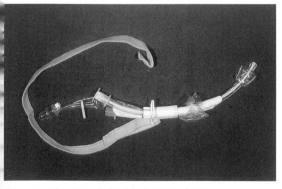

Pharyngolaryngeal double lumen airway.

Tracheal intubation

The ultimate method of airway management for deeply unconscious patients is tracheal intubation. This requires experience and specific equipment. Traditionally the forte of anaesthetists, this skill is now taught to emergency medical staff, specialist nurses, and some ambulance staff. The technique entails flexing the subject's neck, extending the head, exposing the epiglottis with a laryngoscope, lifting the jaw and base of tongue forward to expose the larynx, and inserting a curved tube into the trachea. Inflation of the tracheal cuff isolates the airway and enables ventilation to be performed safely. The risks are of stimulating vomiting in a semiconscious patient, trauma to the mouth and larynx, unilateral bronchial intubation, and unrecognised intubation of the oesophagus.

If tracheal intubation is unsuccessful the procedure should be abandoned without delay and alternative methods of airway control chosen. Techniques for tracheal intubation have been advocated which avoid formal laryngoscopy, but these have a limited success rate even in experienced hands. Blind nasal intubation, digital manipulation of the tube in the laryngopharynx, and transillumination with lighted tube stylets are some methods that have been used.

Pharyngotracheal and oesophageal airways

Several airway devices, more invasive than oropharyngeal airways, have been developed for use by health care professionals who cannot undertake tracheal intubation. They maintain oral and pharyngolaryngeal patency without jaw support and provide a port for mouth or bag ventilation. The pharynx and larynx, however, are highly sensitive areas and stimulation of these areas in semiconscious patients may induce retching, vomiting, and laryngospasm.

The Esophageal Obturator Airway has been popular in the United States for two decades, and has been used in an estimated three million resuscitation attempts. The device consists of a long cuffed tube attached to a facemask. The tube is passed blindly into the oesophagus and the cuff inflated to isolate the oesophagus and stomach from the airway. The oesophageal tube is blocked distally and a series of holes at laryngeal level permit air blown down the tube to pass into the larynx. An alternative device, the Esophageal Gastric Tube Airway, is not sealed at the distal end, thus permitting gastric aspiration or the relief of pressure. A second orifice in the mask is used for ventilation. Problems with the use of oesophageal obturators include the failure to obtain an adequate mask seal, trauma to the oesophagus and stomach, the induction of vomiting sometimes with gastric rupture, and unexpected tracheal intubation.

Alternative cuffed double-lumen devices, also popular in the United States, include the Pharyngo-Tracheal Lumen Airway and the Esophageal Tracheal Combitube. These are inserted blindly into the oropharynx whereupon the pharyngeal balloon is inflated. An assessment is made of which tube has entered the trachea and oesophagus; the tracheal tube is used for ventilation.

The airway at risk

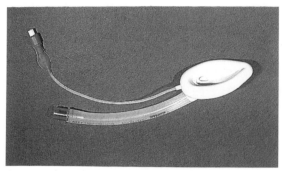

Laryngeal mask airway.

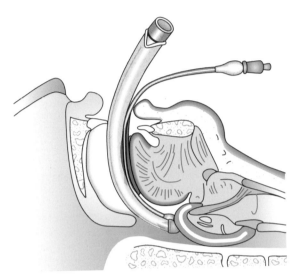

These devices have been reclassified in the 1992 American Heart Association guidelines for cardiopulmonary resuscitation[2] as acceptable and possibly helpful. They have not gained popularity in the United Kingdom, where those who are unable to undertake tracheal intubation generally use oral Guedel airways and mouth-mask or bag-mask ventilation.

Laryngeal mask airway

This innovative airway adjunct, designed in 1983 by Brain,[3] has revolutionised anaesthetic practice in the United Kingdom. A curved tube terminating in a spoon-shaped rubber mask with an inflatable rim, is passed blindly into the hypopharynx to surround and isolate the laryngeal inlet. Five sizes, infant to adult, are available. Competence in laryngeal mask airway insertion can be acquired with minimal training. A level of consciousness between that required for an oral airway and tracheal intubation will allow the laryngeal mask airway to be tolerated. Obstructed ventilation may occur because of laryngospasm or breath-holding, caused by "stimulation" during insertion of the laryngal mask airway, or by displacement or rotation of the mask in the laryngopharynx. Occasionally the epiglottis becomes folded backwards so as to block the laryngeal opening in the mask.

The laryngeal mask airway is used regularly during anaesthesia for both spontaneous and controlled ventilation. The effectiveness of the seal of the cuff in the hypopharynx, in the presence of a full stomach, regurgitation, or vomiting, has still to be fully validated. Because tracheal intubation is not practicable for all prehospital arrests, a strong case can be made for training ambulance crews to use laryngeal mask airway-bag ventilation. Its use by cardiac arrest teams has already been the subject of a favourable multicentre trial.[4]

1 Sellick BA. Cricoid pressure to control regurgitation of stomach contents during induction of anaesthesia. *Lancet* 1961; ii: 404–6.
2 Emergency Cardiac Care Committee and Subcommittees, American Heart Association. Guidelines for cardiopulmonary resuscitation and emergency cardiac care, II: Adult advanced cardiac life support. *JAMA* 1992; **268**: 2199–241.
3 Brain A. The laryngeal mask—A new concept in airway management. *Br J Anaesthesia 1983*; 55: 801–5.
4 Stone BJ, Leach AB, Alexander CA, *et al*. The use of the laryngeal mask airway by nurses during cardiopulmonary resuscitation. Results of a multicentre trial. *Anaesthesia* 1994; **49**: 3–7.

6 RESUSCITATION OF INFANTS AND CHILDREN

David A Zideman

The commonest cause of cardiac arrest in children is a problem with the airway. The resulting difficulties in breathing and the associated hypoxia rapidly cause a severe bradycardia or asystole. In contrast, adults have primary cardiac events resulting in ventricular fibrillation. The poor long term outcome from many cardiac arrests in childhood is related to the severity of cellular anoxia that has to occur before the child's previously healthy heart succumbs. Organs sensitive to anoxia, such as the brain and kidney, may be massively damaged before the heart itself stops. In such cases cardiopulmonary resuscitation may restore cardiac output but the child dies from multisystem failure in the ensuing days or survives with serious neurological damage. Prevention of injury and earlier recognition of illness is clearly a more effective approach in these children.

> **Definitions**
>
> Infant: A child in the first year of life
> Child: From the end of the first year to adulthood

Paediatric basic life support

Early diagnosis and aggressive treatment of respiratory or cardiac insufficiency aimed at avoiding cardiac arrest is the key to improving survival without neurological deficit in seriously ill children. Establishment of a clear airway and oxygenation are the most important actions in paediatric resuscitation. These actions are prerequisites to other forms of treatment.

Resuscitation should begin immediately without waiting for the arrival of equipment. This is essential in infants and children because clearing the airway may be all that is required. Assessment and treatment should proceed simultaneously to avoid losing vital time. As in any resuscitation the airway—breathing—circulation sequence is the most appropriate.

If aspiration of a foreign body is strongly suspected because of sudden onset of severe obstruction of the upper airway the steps outlined in the section on choking should be taken immediately.

Assess responsiveness

Determine responsiveness by speaking loudly, shaking, or pinching gently. If the child is unresponsive shout for help. Move the child only if he or she is in a dangerous location.

Airway

Opening the airway is achieved by tilting the head and supporting the lower jaw. Care must be taken not to overextend the neck (as this may cause the soft trachea to kink and obstruct) and not to press on the soft tissues in the floor of the mouth. Pressure in this area

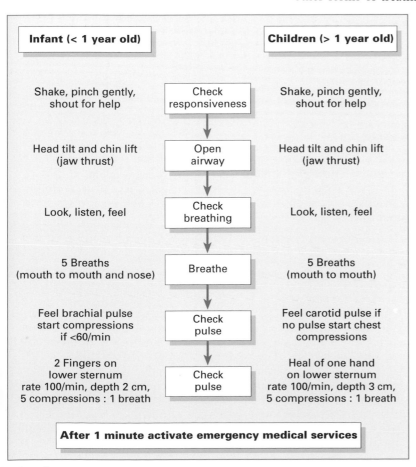

Infant (< 1 year old)		Children (> 1 year old)
Shake, pinch gently, shout for help	Check responsiveness	Shake, pinch gently, shout for help
Head tilt and chin lift (jaw thrust)	Open airway	Head tilt and chin lift (jaw thrust)
Look, listen, feel	Check breathing	Look, listen, feel
5 Breaths (mouth to mouth and nose)	Breathe	5 Breaths (mouth to mouth)
Feel brachial pulse start compressions if <60/min	Check pulse	Feel carotid pulse if no pulse start chest compressions
2 Fingers on lower sternum rate 100/min, depth 2 cm, 5 compressions : 1 breath	Check pulse	Heal of one hand on lower sternum rate 100/min, depth 3 cm, 5 compressions : 1 breath

After 1 minute activate emergency medical services

Resuscitation of infants and children

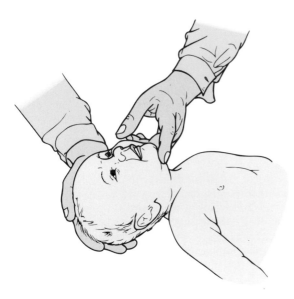

Opening infant airway.

will force the tongue into the airway and cause obstruction. The small infant is an obligatory nose breather so the patency of the nasal passages must be checked and maintained. Maintaining the paediatric airway is a matter of trying various positions until the most satisfactory is found. The rescuer must be flexible and willing to adapt his or her technique.

Breathing

Assess breathing by:
- *Looking* for chest and abdominal movement
- *Listening* at the mouth and nose for breath sounds
- *Feeling* for expired air movement with your cheek.

If the child's chest and abdomen are moving but no air can be heard or felt, the airway is obstructed. Readjust the airway and consider obstruction by a foreign body. Expired air resuscitation must be started immediately if the child is not breathing. With the airway held open, the rescuer should cover the child's mouth (or mouth and nose) with his or her mouth and breathe gently into the child until the chest rises and the child appears to take a deep breath. Minimise gastric distension by optimising the alignment of the airway and giving slow and steady inflations. Five breaths should be delivered, each lasting about 1 to 1·5 seconds.

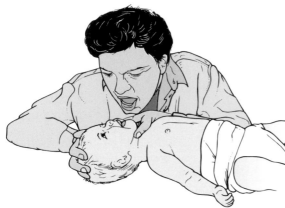

Mouth to mouth and nose ventilation.

Circulation

Check for the presence, rate, and volume of the pulse. The brachial pulse is easiest to feel in infants, the carotid pulse in children. The femoral pulse is an alternative. If the pulse rate is less than 60 beats/min in infants or absent in older children start chest compression without further delay.

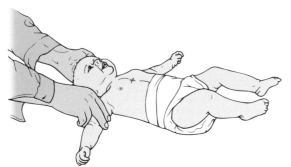

Brachial pulse in infants.

In infants and children the heart lies under the lower third of the sternum. In infants the sternum is compressed with two fingers of one hand, the upper finger being one finger's breadth below an imaginary line joining the nipples. The sternum is compressed about 2 cm. In children the heel of one hand is used at a compression point two fingers' breadth above the xiphoid process. The depth of compression is about 3 cm. In both infants and children the rate should be 100 a minute, and the ratio of compressions to ventilations should be 5:1 irrespective of the number of rescuers. The compression phase should occupy half of the cycle and should be smooth not jerky.

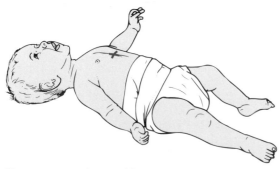

Chest compression position.

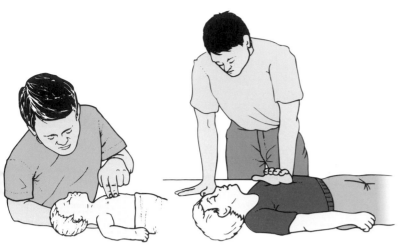

Chest compression in infants and children.

In larger, older children in whom the heel of one hand is found to give an insufficient compression force, the adult two handed method of chest compression can be used (see chapter 1). The compression depth should be 4–5 cm, at a rate of about 80 a minute with a compression to ventilation ratio of 15:2.

Activation of the emergency medical services

Activate energy services after one minute

After one minute of basic life support the emergency medical services must be activated. You should tell the service the rough age of the child. You may be able to carry infants or small children to the telephone, but older children may have to be left. Basic life support must be restarted as soon as possible after telephoning and continued with no further interruptions until help arrives.

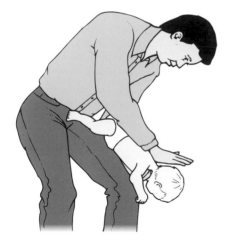

Choking

If airway obstruction due to aspiration of a foreign body is witnessed or strongly suspected special measures to clear the airway must be undertaken. If the child is breathing spontaneously his or her efforts to clear the obstruction should be encouraged. Intervention is necessary only if these attempts are clearly ineffective and respiration is inadequate. Never perform blind finger sweeps of the pharynx as these can impact a foreign body in the larynx. Use measures intended to create a sharp increase in pressure within the chest cavity, an artificial cough.

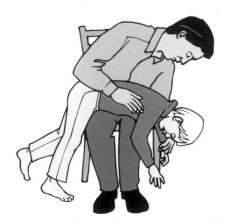

Back blows for choking infants and children.

Back blows—Hold the infant or child in a prone position and deliver five smart blows to the middle of the back between the shoulder blades. The head must be lower than the chest during this manoeuvre. This can be achieved by holding a small infant along the forearm or, for older children, across the thighs while you kneel.

Chest thrusts—With the child in a supine position give five thrusts to the sternum. The technique of chest thrusts is similar to that for chest compressions. The chest thrusts should be sharper and more vigorous than compressions and carried out at a slower rate of 20 a minute.

Check mouth—Remove any visible foreign bodies.

Open airway—Reposition the head by the head tilt and chin lift or jaw thrust manoeuvre and reassess the air entry.

Breathe—Attempt rescue breathing if there are no signs of effective spontaneous respiration or if the airway remains obstructed.

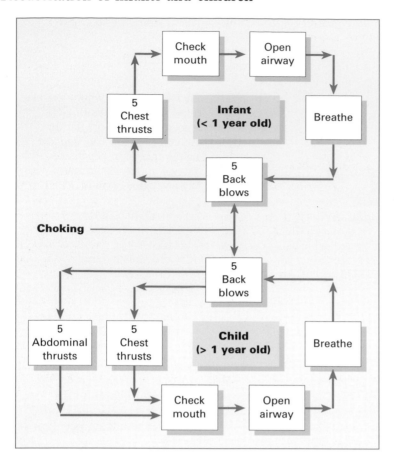

It may be possible to ventilate the child by positive pressure expired air ventilation when the airway is partially obstructed, but care must be taken to ensure that the child exhales most of this artificial ventilation after each breath.

Repeat—If the above procedure is unsuccessful in infants it should be repeated until the airway is cleared and effective respiration established. In children, abdominal thrusts are substituted for chest thrusts after the second round of back blows. Subsequently back blows are combined with chest thrusts or abdominal thrusts in alternate cycles until the airway is cleared.

Abdominal thrusts—In children over 1 year deliver five abdominal thrusts after the second five back blows. Use the upright position (Heimlich manoeuvre) if the child is conscious. Unconscious children should be laid supine and the heel of one hand placed in the middle of the upper abdomen. Five sharp thrusts should be directed upwards towards the diaphragm. Abdominal thrusts are not recommended in infants because they may rupture the abdominal viscera.

Paediatric advanced life support

The use of equipment in paediatric resuscitation is fraught with difficulties. Not only must a wide range of equipment be available to correspond with the variety of sizes of child but the rescuer must also be skilled enough to choose and use the selected equipment. Effective basic life support is a prerequisite for successful advanced life support.

Airway and ventilation management

Airway and ventilation management are particularly important in infants and children after cardiac arrest because respiratory problems are often the cause of the arrest. Oxygen in as high a concentration as possible should be used from the onset in all patients undergoing advanced life support. It should be humified whenever possible.

Airway adjuncts

Use an oropharyngeal (Guedel) airway if the child's airway cannot be maintained adequately by positioning during bag and mask ventilation. A correctly sized airway should extend from the centre of the mouth to the angle of the jaw when laid against the child's face.

Tracheal intubation is the most effective method of securing the airway. The technique facilitates ventilation and oxygenation and prevents pulmonary aspiration of gastric contents. A child's larynx is narrower and shorter than that of any adult, and the epiglottis is relatively longer and more U shaped. The larynx is also in a higher, more anterior and more acutely angled position than in the adult. A straight bladed laryngoscope and plain plastic uncuffed tracheal tubes are therefore used in infants and young children. In children aged over 1 year the appropriate size of tracheal tube can be assessed by the following formula:

$$\text{internal diameter (mm)} = (\text{age in years}/4) + 4$$

Another useful guideline is to use a tube of about the same diameter as the child's little finger or of a size that will just fit into the nostril.

Full term newborn infants usually require a tube of size 3 to 3·5 increasing to a size 4 by 6 to 9 months of age.

Basic life support must not be interrupted for more than 30 seconds. After this interval the child must be reoxygenated before a further attempt at intubation is made.

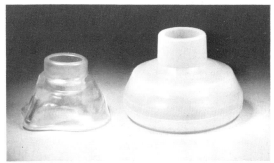

Paediatric masks.

Oxygenation and ventilation adjuncts

A flow meter capable of delivering 15 l/min should be attached to the oxygen supply from either a central wall pipeline or an independent oxygen cylinder. Face masks for mouth to mask or bag valve mask ventilation should be made of soft clear plastic, have a low dead space, and conform to the child's face to form a good seal. Circular facemasks have been found to be more easily used by the inexperienced. The face mask should be attached to a self inflating bag of either 500 ml or 1600 ml capacity. The smaller size has a pressure limiting valve. Occasionally, this may need to be overridden if the child's lungs have poor compliance. The bag valve mask system must be used with a reservoir attachment. This reservoir, together with high flow supplemental oxygen, enables an inspired oxygen concentration of over 90% to be delivered. The T piece and open ended bag system is not recommended for less experienced operators as it requires specialist training.

Management protocols for advanced life support

Asystole

Asystole is the most common arrest rhythm in infancy and childhood. It is the final common pathway of respiratory or circulatory failure. It is usually preceded by an agonal bradycardia.

The diagnosis of asystole is made on electrocardiographic evidence in a pulseless patient. Care must be taken to ensure that the electrocardiograph leads are correctly positioned and attached and that the monitor gain is turned up. The algorithm shows the protocol for managing asystole. Effective basic life support and ventilation with high flow oxygen through a patent airway are prerequisites. The process is simple in that having established a secure airway and intravenous or intraosseous access, 10 μg/kg of adrenaline is administered followed by three minutes of basic life support. If asystole persists then the dose of adrenaline should be raised to 100 μg/kg and repeated every three minutes.

Alkalising agents are of unproved benefit and should be used only after clinical consideration of profound acidosis in patients with respiratory or circulatory arrest if the first dose of adrenaline has been ineffectual. The dose of bicarbonate is 1 mmol/kg given as a single bolus by slow intravenous injection before the second dose of adrenalin. If an alkalising agent is used the cannula must be flushed with normal saline before subsequent infusion of a catecholamine as catecholomines are inactivated by the alkalising agent. Subsequent treatment with alkalising agents should be guided by the blood pH.

A bolus of normal saline should follow the intravenous or intraosseous injection of any drug used in resuscitation, especially if the injection is peripheral. The amount should be 5–20 ml depending on the size of the child. When cardiac arrest has resulted from circulatory failure a larger bolus of fluid should be given if there is no response or a poor response to the initial dose of adrenaline. Examples of such cases are children with hypovolaemia from blood loss, gastroenteritis, etc, or with sepsis when a profound distributive hypovolaemic shock may occur. These children require 20 ml/kg of a crystalloid, such as normal saline or Ringer's lactate, or a colloid, such as 5% human albumin or an artificial colloid. Take care not to overload the venous circulation because an increase in right atrial pressure will decrease coronary perfusion pressure.

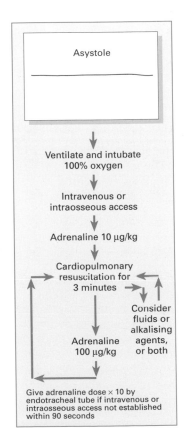

Asystole

Ventilate and intubate
100% oxygen

Intravenous or
intraosseous access

Adrenaline 10 μg/kg

Cardiopulmonary
resuscitation for
3 minutes

Consider
fluids or
alkalising
agents,
or both

Adrenaline
100 μg/kg

Give adrenaline dose × 10 by
endotracheal tube if intravenous or
intraosseous access not established
within 90 seconds

Resuscitation of infants and children

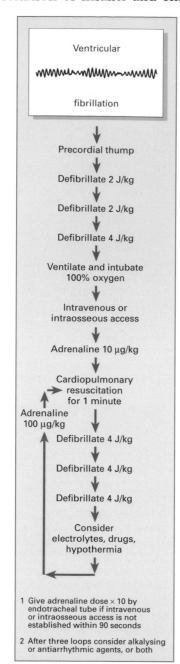

Ventricular fibrillation

↓

Precordial thump

↓

Defibrillate 2 J/kg

↓

Defibrillate 2 J/kg

↓

Defibrillate 4 J/kg

↓

Ventilate and intubate
100% oxygen

↓

Intravenous or
intraosseous access

↓

Adrenaline 10 μg/kg

↓

Cardiopulmonary
resuscitation
for 1 minute

Adrenaline
100 μg/kg

↓

Defibrillate 4 J/kg

↓

Defibrillate 4 J/kg

↓

Defibrillate 4 J/kg

↓

Consider
electrolytes, drugs,
hypothermia

1 Give adrenaline dose × 10 by
endotracheal tube if intravenous
or intraosseous access is not
established within 90 seconds

2 After three loops consider alkalysing
or antiarrhythmic agents, or both

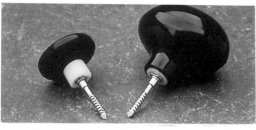

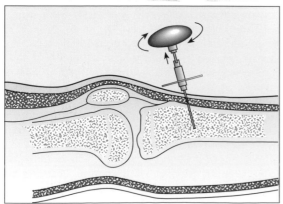

Intraosseous infusion needle. (Cook)

Ventricular fibrillation

Ventricular fibrillation is unusual in children, but it is occasionally seen in cardiothoracic intensive care units or in patients being investigated for congenital heart disease. In other patients there is usually an underlying cause that may need correction before defibrillation is successful—for example, hypothermia, arrhythmia inducing drugs such as tricylic antidepressants, and electrolyte abnormalities such as hypokalaemia. The algorithm shows the protocol for treating ventricular fibrillation and pulseless ventricular tachycardia. In contrast with the treatment of asystole defibrillation takes precedence. A precordial thump can be given and may be effective if the start of ventricular fibrillation was witnessed. The energy dose is 2J/kg rising to 4J/kg if two shocks of the lower dose are ineffective. For defibrillators with stepped current levels the nearest higher step to the current required should be selected. Ventilation and chest compressions should be continued at all times except when shocks are being delivered or the electrocardiogram being studied for evidence of change. Paediatric paddles should be used in children below 10 kg, but in bigger children the larger adult electrode will minimise transthoracic impedance and should be used when the child's thorax is broad enough to permit electrode to chest contact over the entire paddle surface. One paddle should be placed over the apex of the heart and one beneath the right clavicle.

Electromechanical dissociation

As in ventricular fibrillation there may be an underlying remediable cause for electromechanical dissociation (pulseless electrical activity) in children. This cause should be sought while life support continues. The most likely cause for apparent electromechanical dissociation is profound hypovolaemic shock causing impalpable central pulses while there is still electrical activity in the heart. If not treated this rhythm will soon degenerate through agonal bradycardia to asystole. Other underlying causes to consider, especially in trauma, are tension pneumothorax and cardiac tamponade. Although a pulmonary embolism can cause electromechanical dissociation, it is extremely rare in childhood. Metabolic abnormalities such as hypothermia, electrolyte imbalance, and a drug overdose should also be considered.

The algorithm shows the protocol for treating electromechanical dissociation. The process is similar to that for asystole with oxygenation and ventilation accompanying basic life support and adrenaline to support coronary and cerebral perfusion. In view of the likelihood of correctable hypovolaemia, early use of a bolus of 20 ml/kg of crystalloid or colloid is indicated. If fluid replacement is initially unsuccessful cerebral and coronary perfusion should be sustained by ventilation, chest compressions, and adrenaline 100 μg/kg every three minutes while any of the underlying causes suggested are identified and corrected.

Routes of drugs and fluid administration

Venous—Speed is vital when giving drugs and fluid to patients in cardiac arrest. Peripheral venous access in small ill children is notoriously difficult. Central venous access is hazardous in small children and unlikely to provide a more rapid onset of action of drugs than peripheral access. If venous access is already available it should be used. Otherwise peripheral venous access should be attempted. If access is not gained within 90 seconds bone marrow (intraosseous) access should be attempted.

Intraosseous—Intraosseous access is a safe, simple, and rapid means of access for children of all ages and even adults. Resuscitation drugs, fluid, and blood can be safely given through this route and rapidly reach the heart. Complications are uncommon and usually relate to prolonged use or poor technique. Marrow aspirate can be drawn and used to estimate concentrations of haemoglobin, sodium, potassium, chloride, and glucose and venous pH and blood groups.

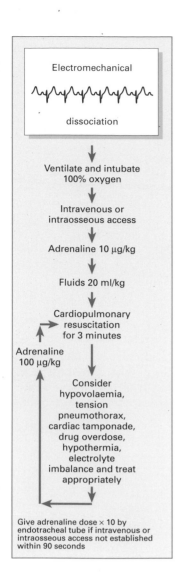

Give adrenaline dose × 10 by endotracheal tube if intravenous or intraosseous access not established within 90 seconds

Endotracheal—If circulatory access is impossible to attain within two to three minutes some drugs, including adrenaline, atropine, and lignocaine, can be given down the tracheal tube. Data from studies on animals and humans suggest that the endotracheal dose of adrenaline should be 10 times the standard dose, but doubts have been cast on the reliability of this route and intravenous or intraosseous access is preferable.

Drug doses and equipment sizes

An important problem in managing cardiac arrest in children is the correct estimation of drug and fluid doses and equipment sizes. There are two systems in current use. The first uses a calculation based on length and a specifically designed tape measure (the Broselow tape).[1] The other uses a length-weight-age nomogram chart (the Oakley chart).[2 3] It is important to become familiar with one system.

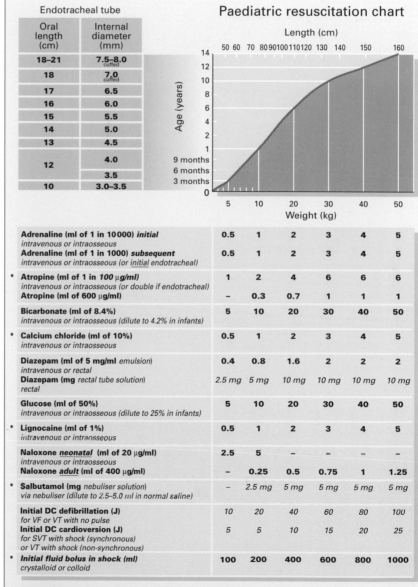

1 Luten RC, Wears RL, Broselow J, Zaritsky A, Barnett TM, Lee T. Length-based endotracheal tube and emergency equipment selection in paediatrics. *Ann Emerg Med* 1992; **2**: 900–4.
2 Oakley PA. Inaccuracy and delay in decision making in paediatric resuscitation and a proposed reference chart to reduce error. *BMJ* 1988; **297**: 817–9.
3 Oakley PA, Phillips B, Molyneux E, Mackway-Jones K. Paediatric resuscitation. *BMJ* 1994; **306**: 1613.

Further reading

European Resuscitation Council. Guidelines for paediatric resuscitation. *Resuscitation* 1994; **27**: 91–105.
European Resuscitation Council. Guidelines for paediatric resuscitation. *BMJ* 1994; **308**: 1349–55.
APLS Working Group. *Advanced paediatric life support. The practical approach.* London: BMJ Publishing Group, 1994.
Zideman DA. Paediatric resuscitation. In: Baskett PJF, ed. *Resuscitation handbook.* 2nd ed. London: Wolfe Publishing, 1993: 111–20.

7 RESUSCITATION IN PREGNANCY

G A D Rees, B A Willis

Acute causes of 154 maternal deaths out of 238 deaths in pregnancy

Cause	Total no of deaths	No of deaths by subgroup
Haemorrhage:	83	
Uteroplacental		41
Aneurysm or Iatrogenic		6
Cerebrovascular associated with:		
pre-eclampsia/eclampsia		14
non-obstetric		22
Embolism	35	
Pulmonary		24
Amniotic fluid		11
Cardiac	19	
Ischaemic heart disease		6
Other		4
Congenital heart disease		9
Anaesthesia	4	
Failed intubation		1
Pulmonary aspiration		1
Spinal anaesthesia		1
Postoperative hypoxia		1
Status epilepticus	9	
Unknown cause	4	

(From *Confidential Enquiries into Maternal Deaths in the UK 1998–1990*)

Cardiac arrest occurs only about once in every 30 000 late pregnancies, but survival from such an event is exceptional. The most recent report on maternal mortality shows that most deaths are due to acute causes so all staff directly or indirectly concerned in obstetric care need to be trained in resuscitation skills.[1]

Factors peculiar to pregnancy that weight the balance against survival include anatomical changes that make it difficult to maintain a clear airway and perform intubation; pathological changes such as laryngeal oedema; physiological factors such as increased oxygen consumption; and an increased likelihood of pulmonary aspiration. In the third trimester, however, the most important factor of all is compression of the inferior vena cava by the gravid uterus when the woman lies supine. This impairs venous return and withstands the most competent efforts at resuscitation.

Anatomical features relevant to difficult intubation or ventilation

Difficult intubation:
  Full dentition
  Large breasts
  Oedema or obesity of neck
  Supraglottic oedema
  Flared ribcage
  Raised diaphragm

Physiological changes in late pregnancy relevant to cardiopulmonary resuscitation

Respiratory:
  Increased ventilation
  Increased oxygen demand
  Reduced chest compliance
  Reduced functional residual capacity

Cardiovascular:
  Increased cardiac output

Gastrointestinal:
  Incompetent gastro-oesophageal
    (cardiac) sphincter
  Increased intragastric pressure
  Increased risk of regurgitation

A speedy response is essential. Once respiratory or cardiac arrest has been diagnosed the patient must be positioned appropriately and basic life support started immediately. Basic life support must be continued while venous access is secured, any obvious causal factors such as hypovolaemia are corrected, and the equipment, drugs, and staff for advanced life support are assembled.

Basic life support

Airway

A clear airway must be quickly established and then maintained. Suction should be used to aspirate vomit, badly fitting dentures and other foreign bodies should be removed from the mouth, and an airway should be inserted. These procedures should all be performed with the patient supine or inclined laterally with the uterus displaced as described below.

Specific difficulties in pregnant patients

Airway
- Patient inclined laterally (or with uterus displaced if supine) for:
  - Suction aspiration
  - Removing dentures or foreign bodies
  - Inserting airways

Breathing
- Greater oxygen requirement
- Reduced chest compliance
- More difficult to see rise and fall of chest
- More risk of regurgitation and aspiration

Circulation
- External chest compression difficult because:
  - Ribs flared
  - Diaphragm raised
  - Patient obese
  - Breasts hypertrophied
  - Supine position causes inferior vena caval compression by the gravid uterus

---

Breathing

In the absence of adequate respiration intermittent positive pressure ventilation must be started once the airway has been cleared; mouth to mouth, mouth to nose, or mouth to airway ventilation should be carried out until a bag and mask are available; ventilation should then be continued with 100% oxygen by using a reservoir bag. Because of the increased risk of regurgitation and pulmonary aspiration of gastric contents in late pregnancy, cricoid pressure should be applied until the airway is protected by a cuffed tracheal tube.

Ventilation is made more difficult by the increased oxygen requirements and reduced chest compliance that occurs in pregnancy, the latter due to rib flaring and diaphragmatic splinting by the abdominal contents. Observing the rise and fall of the chest in such patients is also more difficult.

Circulation

Circulatory arrest is diagnosed by the absence of a palpable pulse in a large artery (carotid or femoral). Chest compression at a rate of 80 a minute must be started immediately. One inflation should be given after every five compressions if there are two rescuers or two after every 15 compressions if there is a single rescuer.

Chest compression of pregnant women is rendered difficult by flared ribs, raised diaphragm, obesity, and breast hypertrophy. In the supine position an additional factor is compression of the inferior vena cava by the gravid uterus, which impairs venous return and so reduces cardiac output; all attempts at resuscitation will be futile unless the compression is relieved. This can be achieved either by placing the patient in an inclined lateral position by using a wedge or by displacing the uterus manually.

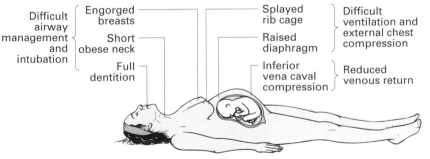

Difficult airway management and intubation
- Engorged breasts
- Short obese neck
- Full dentition

Splayed rib cage / Raised diaphragm — Difficult ventilation and external chest compression

Inferior vena caval compression — Reduced venous return

The Cardiff resuscitation wedge

Effective forces for chest compression can be generated with patients inclined at angles up to 30°, but because of anatomical changes pregnant women tend to roll into a full lateral position when inclined laterally at angles greater than this, making chest compression difficult. The Cardiff resuscitation wedge was based on these observations. It was designed to be portable but substantial enough to withstand resuscitative efforts. The wedge is made from plywood and laminated with plastic for easy cleaning. The position of the patient permits good access and enables the patient's head to be positioned by pillows for intubation and insertion of a central venous line. In studies with a manikin on the Cardiff resuscitation wedge mouth to mouth ventilation and chest compression were as effective in the laterally inclined position as in the supine.[2]

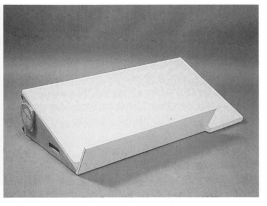

Cardiff resuscitation wedge.

Resuscitation in pregnancy

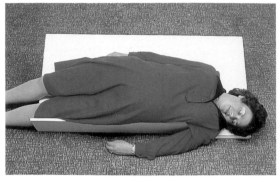

Cardiff resuscitation wedge.

An alternative technique with the lateral position is the "human wedge" where one person relieves caval compression and provides a position stable and firm enough to permit basic life support.

Manual displacement

If some form of wedge is not available the patient should be placed supine on a hard surface to permit conventional chest compression. An assistant must, however, move the uterus off the inferior vena cava by bimanually lifting it to the left and towards the patient's head.

Advanced life support

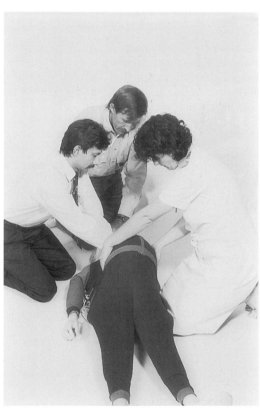

Manual displacement of the uterus.

Intubation

Tracheal intubation should be carried out as soon as facilities and skill are available. A short obese neck and full breasts due to pregnancy may make inserting the laryngoscope into the mouth difficult. The use of a laryngoscope with its blade mounted at more than 90° (Polio or adjustable blade) or demounting the blade from the handle during its insertion into the mouth may help.

Intubation usually follows a period of mouth to mouth or bag and mask ventilation, which is best undertaken without pillows under the head and with the head and neck fully extended. The position for intubation, however, requires at least one pillow flexing the neck with the head extended on the neck. The pillow removed to facilitate initial ventilation must therefore be kept at hand to position the head and neck for intubation.

Defibrillation and drugs

Defibrillation and administration of drugs should be in accordance with the recommendations of the European Resuscitation Council; no special modifications are needed for a pregnant patient.[3]

Caesarian section

Caesarian section is not merely a last ditch attempt to save the life of the fetus but plays an important part in the resuscitation of the mother. This is attested to by the many reports of successful resuscitation after prompt surgical intervention. The probable mechanism for the favourable outcome is that occlusion of the inferior vena cava is relieved completely by emptying the uterus, whereas it is relieved only partially by using the lateral position.

The speed at which surgical delivery is carried out is critical in determining the outcome for both mother and fetus. After cardiac arrest, non-pregnant adults suffer irreversible brain damage from anoxia within 3–4 minutes, but pregnant women become hypoxic more quickly. Although there is evidence that the fetus can tolerate prolonged periods of hypoxia, the outlook for the neonate is optimised by immediate caesarian section.

If maternal cardiac arrest occurs in the labour ward, operating theatre, or casualty department and basic and advanced life support are not successful within five minutes, the uterus should be emptied by surgical intervention. Cardiopulmonary resuscitation must be continued throughout the operation and afterwards as this improves the prognosis for mother and child. After successful delivery both mother and infant should be transferred to their appropriate intensive care units as soon as clinical conditions permit so that their intensive management can be continued.

The key factor for successful resuscitation in late pregnancy is that all nursing and medical staff concerned with obstetric care should be trained in cardiopulmonary resuscitation.

Retention of cardiopulmonary resuscitation skills has been shown to be poor, particularly in staff such as midwives and obstetricians, who have little opportunity to practise them. Regular short periods of practice on a manikin are therefore essential.

Members of the public and the ambulance service also should be aware of the additional problems associated with resuscitation in late pregnancy. The training of ambulance staff in cardiopulmonary resuscitation in late pregnancy is of particular importance as paramedics are likely to be the primary responders to community obstetric emergency calls in the future.

1 Hibbard BM, Anderson MM, Drife JO *et al*. *Report on confidential enquiries into maternal deaths in the United Kingdom 1988–1990*. London: HMSO, 1994.
2 Rees GAD, Willis BA. Resuscitation in late pregnancy. *Anaesthesia* 1988; **43**: 347–9.
3 European Resuscitation Council. *Resuscitation* 1992; **24**: 111–21.

8 RESUSCITATION AT BIRTH

A D Milner

High risk deliveries

Delivery
Fetal distress
Reduced fetal
    movement
Abnormal
    presentation
Prolapsed cord
Antepartum
    haemorrhage
Meconium staining
    of liquor
High forceps
Ventouse
Caesarean section
    under general
    anaesthetic

Maternal
Severe pregnancy induced hypertension
Heavy sedation
Drug addiction
Diabetes mellitus
Chronic illness

Fetal
Multiple pregnancy
Preterm (<34/52)
Post-term (>42/52)
Small for dates
Rhesus
    isoimmunisation
Hydramnios and
    oligohydramnios
Abnormal baby

The priority for all those responsible for the care of babies at birth must be to ensure that adequate resuscitation facilities are available. Sadly, some babies have irreversible brain damage by the time of delivery, but it is unacceptable that any damage should occur after delivery because equipment is inadequate or staff insufficiently trained.

All babies known to be at increased risk should be delivered in a unit with full respiratory support facilities and must always be attended by a doctor who is skilled in resuscitation and solely responsible for the care of that baby. Whenever possible there should also be a trained assistant who can provide additional help if necessary. The list of causes of increased risk is fairly long. Such babies make up about a quarter of all deliveries and about two thirds of those requiring resuscitation; the remaining one third are babies born after a normal uneventful labour who have no apparent risk factors. Staff on labour wards must therefore always be prepared to provide adequate resuscitation until further help can be obtained.

Equipment

The padded platform on which the baby is resuscitated can either be flat or have a head down tilt. It can be mounted on the wall or kept on a trolley provided that one is available for each delivery area. It is essential that there should be an overhead heater with an output of 300–500 watts mounted about 1 metre above the platform. This must have a manual control as servo systems are slow to set up and likely to malfunction when the baby's skin is wet. These heaters are essential as even in environments of 20–24°C the core temperature of an asphyxiated wet baby can drop by 5°C in as many minutes. Facilities must be available for manual face mask resuscitation, tracheal tube resuscitation, and catheterisation of the umbilical vein. Additional equipment should include an overhead light, a clock with a second hand, suction equipment, a stethoscope, and preferably an electrocardiographic monitor.

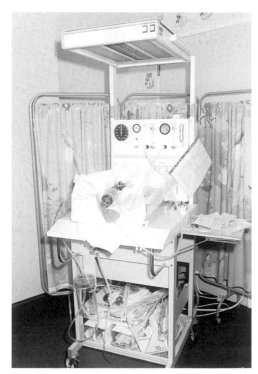

Neonatal resuscitation trolley.

Resuscitation equipment

Padded shelf/resuscitation trolley
Overhead heater
Overhead light
Oxygen supply
Clock
Stethoscope
Airway pressure manometer and pressure relief valve
Face mask
Oropharyngeal airways 00 + 0
Resuscitation system (face mask/T piece/bag and mask)
Suction catheters (sized 5, 8, 10 FG)
Mechanical and/or manual suction with double trap
Two laryngoscopes with spare blades
Endotraceal tubes 2, 2.5, 3, 3.5, and 4 mm, introducer
Umbilical vein catheterisation set
Umbilical artery catheterisation set
2, 10 And 20 ml syringes with needles
ECG and transcutaneous oxygen saturation monitor
Note: capnometers are a strongly recommended optional extra

Procedure at delivery

Pharyngeal suction

Rarely necessary unless amniotic fluid stained with meconium or blood

Can delay onset of spontaneous respiration for long time if suction aggressive

Not recommended by direct mouth suction or oral mucus extractors since congenital infection with HIV recognised

In most units it is standard policy during labour to suck out the pharynx as soon as the face appears by using a suction catheter. This is almost always unnecessary, unless the amniotic fluid is stained with meconium or blood. Aggressive pharyngeal suction can delay the onset of spontaneous respiration for a considerable time. Once the baby is delivered the attendant should wipe any excess fluid off the baby with a warm towel to reduce evaporative heat loss at the same time examining the child for major external congenital abnormalities, such as spina bifida and severe microcephaly. Most babies will start breathing during this period as the median time until the onset of spontaneous respiration is only 10 seconds. They can then be handed to their parents. If necessary the baby can be encouraged to breathe by skin stimulation, for example flicking the baby's feet; those not responding must be transferred immediately to the resuscitation area.

Resuscitation procedure

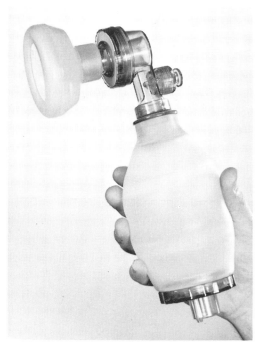
Bag-valve-mask device.

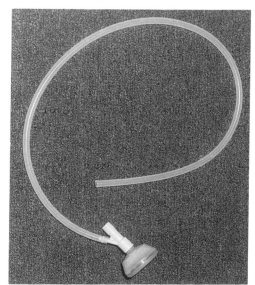
Face mask and tubing.

Check first for respiratory efforts. If these are present, even vigorous, but producing no tidal exchange the airway is obstructed. This can often be overcome by extending the baby's neck. If the baby has choanal atresia or Pierre Robin syndrome (cleft palate and micrognathia) obstruction will continue until an airway is inserted.

If respiratory efforts are feeble or totally absent count the heart rate for 10–15 seconds with a stethoscope. When the heart rate is over 80 beats/min it is sufficient to repeat skin stimulation and if this fails to proceed to face mask resuscitation.

Face mask resuscitation

Only face masks consisting of a soft continuous ring provide an adequate seal. Most standard devices for manual resuscitation of the neonate fail to produce adequate tidal exchange when the pressure limiting device is unimpeded. Thus a satisfactory outcome almost always depends on the inflation pressure stimulating the baby to make inspiratory efforts (Head's paradoxical reflex). This poor performance is related to the short inspiratory time (one third to half a second) provided by the devices. Tidal exchange can be increased by using a 500 ml rather than a standard 250 ml reservoir, which allows inflation pressure to be maintained for one second.

More satisfactory tidal exchange can be achieved by bleeding oxygen directly into the face mask at 4–6 l/minute and occluding the outlet from the face mask as if it were an endotracheal T piece. It is obviously essential to incorporate a pressure valve into the inspiratory lines so that the pressure cannot exceed 30 cm H_2O. The baby's lungs can then be inflated at rates of about 30 a minute, allowing 1 second for each part of the cycle. Listen to the baby's chest after 5–10 inflations to check that there is bilateral air entry and that the heart rate is satisfactory. If the heart rate falls below 80 beats/min proceed immediately to tracheal intubation.

Tracheal intubation

Most non-anaesthetists find a straight bladed laryngoscope preferable for performing intubation. This must be held in the left hand and the baby's neck gently extended, if necessary by the assistant. Pass the laryngoscope down, making sure that it is in the mid-line, until the epiglottis comes into view. The tip of the blade can then be positioned either proximal to or immediately over the epiglottis so that the cords are brought into view. Gentle backwards pressure may need to be applied over the larynx at this stage. As the airway tends to be filled with fluid the upper airway may have to be cleared with the suction catheter held in the right hand.

Once the cords are visible pass the tracheal tube with the right hand and remove the laryngoscope blade, taking care that this does not displace the tube out of the larynx. Then attach the tracheal tube either to a T piece system incorporating a 30–40 cm H_2O blow off valve in the inspiratory line or to a neonatal manual resuscitation device. If a T piece is used maintain the initial inflation pressure for two to three

Resuscitation at birth

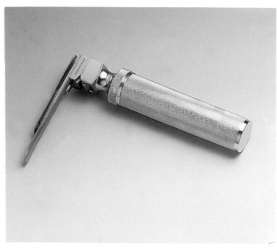

Straight bladed laryngoscope.

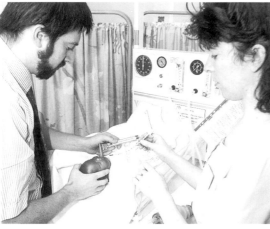

Neonatal intubation.

seconds, which will help lung expansion. The baby can subsequently be ventilated at a rate of 30 a minute, allowing about 1 second for each inflation.

Inspect the chest during the first few inflations, looking for evidence of chest wall movement, and confirm by auscultation that oxygen is entering both lungs. If there is no air entry the most likely cause is that the tracheal tube is lying in the oesophagus. If this is suspected remove the tube immediately and reintubate. If auscultation shows that oxygen is entering one lung only, usually the right, try withdrawing the tube by 1 cm while listening over the left lung. If this leads to dramatic improvement the tip of the endotracheal tube was lying in the right main bronchus. If there is no improvement the possible causes include pneumothorax, diaphragmatic hernia, or pleural effusion.

Severe bradycardia

If the heart rate falls below 30 beats/min chest compression must be started by pressing over the junction of the lower and middle third of the sternum with the tips of two fingers or by placing a hand round the chest and compressing it between the thumb and fingers at a rate of 100–120 compressions a minute. This will achieve about three compressions for every ventilation. If there is no dramatic improvement within 10–15 seconds the umbilical vein should be catheterised with a 5 French gauge catheter. This is best achieved by transecting the cord 2–3 cm away from the abdominal skin and inserting a catheter until there is free flow of blood up the catheter. The baby should then be given 3 mmol of sodium bicarbonate per kg of body weight over two to three minutes. This is best provided by mixing 8·4% solution with an equal volume of 10% dextrose, injecting a total of 20 ml to a term baby and 10 ml to a small baby, while continuing chest compressions and intermittent positive pressure ventilation. Those who fail to respond or who are in asystole require 1 ml of 1 in 10 000 solution of adrenaline. This can be given either intravenously or injected directly down the tracheal tube.

It is reasonable to continue with this regimen for 20 minutes, even in those who are born in apparent asystole, provided that a foetal heart beat was noted within 15 minutes of delivery. Resuscitation efforts should not be continued beyond half an hour unless the baby is making at least intermittent respiratory efforts.

Resuscitation procedure

Intravenous naloxone (100 μg/kg) should be given to all babies who become pink and have an obviously satisfactory circulation after resuscitation but fail to start adequate respiratory efforts. There is often a history of recent maternal opiate sedation. Alternatively, the naloxone can be given down the tracheal tube. Some authorities recommend that an additional 200 μg should be given intramuscularly to prevent relapse. Naloxone must not be given to infants of mothers addicted to opiates as this will provoke severe withdrawal symptoms.

Meconium aspiration

Direct laryngoscopy should be carried out immediately after birth whenever there is meconium staining. If this reveals meconium in the pharynx and trachea, intubate the child immediately and attach the side port of the tracheal tube to the suction source. Suck up the free fluid while the endotracheal tube is removed and then reintubate. Provided the baby's heart rate remains about 60 beats/min this procedure can be repeated until meconium is no longer recovered. The use of direct mouth suction or even oral mucous extractors has been discouraged since infection with HIV was established as occurring congenitally.

Babies with a gestation of more than 32 weeks do not differ from full term babies in their requirement for resuscitation. At less than this gestation they may have a lower morbidity and mortality if a more active intervention policy is adopted. There is, however, no evidence that a rigid policy whereby all babies with a gestation of less that 28 or

---

Drugs

1 : 10 000 adrenalin
Naloxone hydrochloride (200 μg/ml)
Alkalising agent (sodium bicarbonate,
    Tham, or mixture)
Sodium chloride 0.9%
Dextrose (10–20%)
Immediate access to plasma expanders
Access to group O rhesus negative blood
Facilities for ECG and transcutaneous
    saturation are strongly recommended

---

30 weeks are routinely intubated leads to improved outcome. Indeed, unless the operator is extremely skilful, intervention may produce severe hypoxia in a previously lively pink baby and produce conditions that may well predispose to intraventricular haemorrhage. A reasonable compromise would therefore seem to be to start face mask resuscitation at 15–30 seconds unless the baby has entirely adequate respiratory efforts and to proceed to intubation if the baby has not achieved satisfactory respiratory efforts by 30–60 seconds.

9 RESUSCITATION IN HOSPITAL

T R Evans

A patient suffering a cardiac arrest in a British hospital has a one in three chance of initial successful resuscitation, a one in five chance of leaving hospital alive, and a one in seven chance of still being alive one year later. Younger patients and those who are being nursed in a specialist area at the time of cardiac arrest (such as a cardiac care unit or accident and emergency department) have a considerably better outlook, with about twice the chance of surviving one year.

Any patient suffering a cardiopulmonary arrest in hospital has the right to expect the maximum chance of survival as staff should be appropriately trained and equipped in all aspects of resuscitation.

A hospital may be considered as being divided into three types of area:
● Specialist areas—cardiac care, intensive care, accident and emergency, operating theatres, and specialist intervention areas such as cardiac catheterisation laboratories and endoscopy units
● General areas—wards and departments such as physiotherapy, outpatients, and radiology
● The overall concourse areas of the hospital.

In the specialist areas a fully equipped resuscitation trolley should always be on site with staff who are trained in advanced life support and defibrillation.

It is desirable for every ward to have its own defibrillator and resuscitation trolley, with a trained nurse on the ward able to defibrillate by using either a manual or automated external defibrillator. The minimum requirement is for one defibrillator and one trolley on each clinical floor of the hospital.

Cardiac arrest can occur anywhere else in the hospital so as many of the clerical, administrative, and other support staff as possible should be trained in basic life support, to render immediate assistance while awaiting the cardiac arrest team.

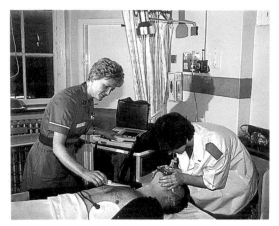

Cardiac arrest on the ward; one nurse ventilates the patient while another prepares an automated defibrillator.

Training of staff in cardiopulmonary resuscitation

> **The Advanced Life Support course of the Resuscitation Council (UK) teaches the skills required of members of the hospital cardiac arrest team**

Medical and nursing staff should possess the skills that they are likely to have to practise in an emergency. All members (or potential members) of the resuscitation team and all staff working in specialist units should be trained in advanced life support techniques and, whenever possible, have successfully completed an advanced life support provider course approved by the Resuscitation Council (UK). They should attend refresher courses at regular intervals.

Staff working in other areas where cardiac arrest is rare should be regularly trained and retrained in basic life support and in how to call the resuscitation team.

The resuscitation committee

> **All health districts should have a multidisciplinary resuscitation committee**

Every hospital should have a resuscitation committee as recommended in the 1987 Royal College of Physicians' report on resuscitation from cardiopulmonary arrest. Its composition will vary slightly from hospital to hospital, but specialists in cardiology and/or general medicine, anaesthesia and critical care, accident and emergency, and paediatrics should normally form the nucleus of the committee, together with the resuscitation training officer, nursing staff representatives, pharmacists, telephonists, and representatives of the administrative and support staff such as porters who transport the cardiac arrest trolley. The committee should ensure that hospital staff are appropriately and adequately trained, that there is sufficient resuscitation equipment in good working order throughout the hospital, and that adequate training facilities are available. The minutes of the committee's meetings should be sent to the medical director or appropriate medical executive or advisory committee of the hospital and should highlight any dangerous or deficient areas of practice such as lack of equipment or properly trained staff. In hospitals where there are postgraduate deans and/or tutors, they should be ex-officio members of the committee to facilitate liaison on training matters and ensure that adequate time and money is set aside to allow junior doctors to receive training in resuscitation.

The resuscitation committee should receive a regular audit of procedures for cardiac arrest, hold audit meetings, and take remedial action if it seems necessary.

The resuscitation training officer

The resuscitation training officer plays a vital part in ensuring that staff are suitably trained. He or she must be highly proficient at basic and advanced life support procedures for adults and preferably also for children. The officer should be directly responsible to the chair of the resuscitation committee and receive its full backing in carrying out his or her role as defined by that committee. At the time of writing there are only about 140 officers in post, indicating that many hospitals have yet to make such an appointment. The British Heart Foundation has been instrumental in "pump priming" new posts, but hospitals must be prepared subsequently to cover the salary and associated training costs from their own budgets.

It is reasonable to expect a training officer to be a Resuscitation Council (UK) advanced life support instructor; many are instructors in paediatric resuscitation as well. It is desirable that they should also hold an advanced trauma life support provider certificate, although currently only doctors can train as instructors.

Resuscitation training officers come from a variety of backgrounds: coronary care, intensive care, or accident and emergency nurses; operating department assistants; and some paramedics from the statutory ambulance service.

Adequate office space, secretarial help, and a dedicated training room for resuscitation are essential for the officer to perform his or her duties efficiently. As well as conducting the inhospital audit of resuscitation, he or she should be encouraged to undertake research studies. Doctors, nurses, and managers have not always recognised the crucial importance of having a resuscitation training officer and have tended to give the appointment low priority for funding. It is hoped that with the medical Royal Colleges taking a greater interest in resuscitation training for doctors approval of junior training posts will be made dependent on a resuscitation training officer being appointed.

It is recommended that the Royal College of Physicians' 1987 report should be implemented in full in all hospitals.

All hospitals should have a unique telephone number to be used in cases of suspected cardiac arrest. This number should be displayed prominently on every telephone and should sound an alarm in the hospital telephone exchange, giving the call equal priority with a fire alarm call. Because the person instigating the call may not know exactly what location they are calling from the telephone should indicate this also—for example, cardiac arrest Marsden Ward sixth floor. By pressing a single button in the telephone exchange all the cardiac arrest bleeps should sound and indicate the location of the cardiac arrest.

The local resuscitation committee should determine the composition of the cardiac arrest team, which may include a registrar or senior house officer in medicine and anaesthesia, another junior doctor, nursing staff, and sometimes an operating department assistant. In multistorey hospitals those carrying the cardiac arrest bleep must have an override facility to commandeer the lifts.

The training officer must ensure that after each attempt at resuscitation the necessary documentation is adequate and accurately

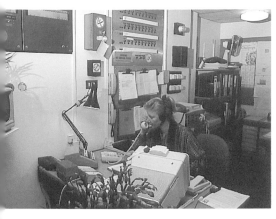

Switchboard operator receiving a cardiac arrest call.

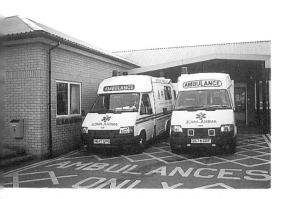

The resuscitation room in the accident and emergency department should be near the ambulance entrance.

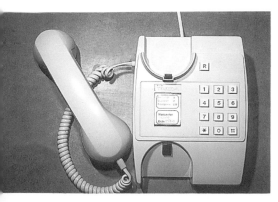

The emergency number to call the cardiac arrest team should be clearly visible on all telephones and known to all members of staff.

completed, preferably in "Utstein format." Usually the nursing staff will check and restock the resuscitation trolley.

Whenever possible the senior doctor in charge should debrief the team whether the resuscitation attempt has been successful or not. Problems should be frankly discussed. If any member of staff is especially distressed a counselling facility should be made available through the occupational health or psychological medicine department.

The resuscitation training room

Every hospital should have a room or dedicated area fully equipped with resuscitation manikins, arrhythmia simulators, intubation trainers, and other training aids.

Do not resuscitate (DNR) orders

For some patients attempts at cardiopulmonary resuscitation are inappropriate, usually because of the terminal nature of the illness or the futility of the attempt. Every hospital's resuscitation committee should agree a "Do not resuscitate" policy with its ethics committee (see chapter 17). In some cases it will be appropriate to discuss the suitability of attempting resuscitation with a patient or his or her representatives in the light of the patient's diagnosis, the probability of success, and the likely quality of life subsequently. When a competent person has expressed their views on resuscitation in an advance directive or living will these wishes should usually be respected. Do not resuscitate orders must be clearly documented in the medical and nursing notes and be subjected to renewal at regular predetermined intervals. In the absence of a standing Do not resuscitate order, cardiopulmonary resuscitation must be started on every patient irrespective of disease or age. Guidelines on the application of such policies have been published by the BMA jointly with the Royal College of Nursing and also by the Royal College of Physicians.

Intermediate life support

It may be appropriate to train a group of responders, usually nursing staff from critical care, to respond to cardiac arrest calls with automated external defibrillators and, perhaps, laryngeal mask airways. Early defibrillation is the way to improved survival; ideally patients should be defibrillated before the cardiac arrest team arrives.

Medical students

All undergraduate medical students should be taught basic life support in the first preclinical year and their skills should be refreshed frequently thereafter. Advanced life support techniques should be taught during the clinical course, hopefully leading to advanced life support provider certificate from the Resuscitation Council (UK).

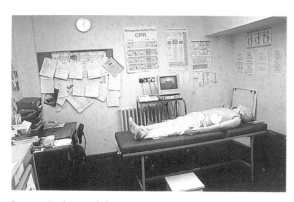
Resuscitation training room.

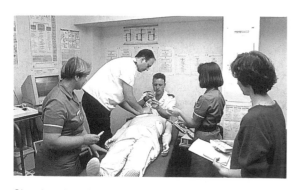
Simulated cardiac arrest training.

Further reading

Royal College of Physicians. Resuscitation from cardiopulmonary arrest: training and organization. *J R Coll Physicians Lond* 1987; **21**: 1–8.

Tunstall-Pedoe H, Bailey L, Chamberlain DA, Marsden AK, Ward ME, Zideman DA. Survey of 3765 cardiopulmonary resuscitations in British hospitals (the BRESUS study): methods and overall results. *BMJ* 1992; **304**: 1347–51.

Chamberlain DA, Cummins RO, Abramson N, Allen M, *et al*. Recommended guidelines for uniform reporting of data from out-of-hospital cardiac arrest: the 'Utstein style'. *Resuscitation* 1991; **22**: 1–26.

Williams R. The 'do not resuscitate' decision; guidelines for policy in the adult. *J R Coll Physicians Lond* 1993; **27**: 139–40.

Royal College of Nursing, British Medical Association. *Cardiopulmonary resuscitation*. London: RCN, 1993.

10 RESUSCITATION IN THE AMBULANCE SERVICE

Andrew K Marsden, Richard Vincent

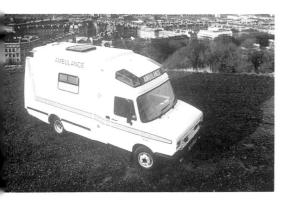

Sudden death outside hospital is common; in England alone more than 50 000 medically unattended deaths occur each year. The survival of countless victims of acute myocardial infarction, primary cardiac arrhythmia, trauma, or vascular catastrophe is threatened through lack of urgent care while they are remote from the skills and facilities of a hospital service. The case for providing prompt and effective resuscitation at the scene of an emergency is overwhelming, but only in the past few years has it begun to receive the attention it deserves.

Development of resuscitation ambulances

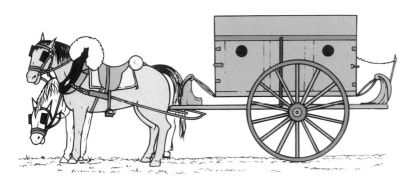

The concept of delivering care at the scene of the emergency was first developed by Baron von Larrey, a young French army surgeon who, in 1792, devised a light vehicle that bore the military surgeons and their equipment right up to the front battle lines of the Napoleonic wars. Larrey's walking carts or horse drawn *ambulances volantes* ("flying ambulances") were the forerunners of the highly sophisticated mobile intensive care units of today.

The delivery of emergency care to patients before admission to hospital was pioneered in Europe in the late 1960s. Pilot schemes, notable among which was Professor Frank Pantridge's mobile coronary care unit in Belfast in 1966, showed that resuscitation vehicles crewed by *medical or nursing staff* could bring effective treatment to the victims of sudden illness or trauma.[1]

The use of emergency vehicles carrying only *paramedic staff*—either in telephone contact with the hospital or acting entirely without supervision—was explored in the early 1970s, most extensively in the United States. Under the Medic 1 scheme started in Seattle in 1970 by Dr Leonard Cobb, the tenders of a highly coordinated fire service can reach an emergency in any part of the city within four minutes. All fire fighters were trained in basic life support and defibrillation and were supported by well equipped Medic 1 ambulances crewed by paramedics who have received at least 12 months' full time training in emergency care.

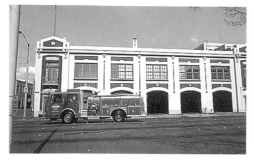

The emergency medical services in Seattle are supported by an extensive community resuscitation programme.

In the United Kingdom the development of civilian paramedic schemes has been slow. The Brighton experiment in ambulance training began in 1971[2] and schemes in other centres followed independently over the next few years. But rapid progress in paramedic training was hindered by the hesitation of hospital staff to accept the role of prehospital care and by the initial caution of the Department of Health and Social Security in supporting developments in this field. It was only due to individual enthusiasm (by pioneers like Baskett, Chamberlain, and Ward) and private donations for equipment that any progress was made. After suggestions in the Miller report (1966–7) and the recognition by the Department of Health of the value of prehospital care, a pilot course on extended training in ambulance aid was launched

Emergencies in which well trained paramedic crew can play vital part

- Life threatening arrhythmias
- Respiratory arrest
- Hypovolaemic shock (internal haemorrhage; trauma)
- Uncomplicated myocardial infarction
- Severe left ventricular failure
- Airway obstruction
- Severe bronchospasm
- Hypoglycaemia
- Head injury
- Drug overdose
- Obstetric emergencies

by the National Staff Committee and formalised by the NHS training authority in 1987. Three years later, after industrial action within the ambulance service, the then minister of health, Kenneth Clarke, pronounced that extended trained paramedics should be involved with every emergency ambulance call and funding was made available to provide each front line ambulance with a defibrillator. In Scotland because of an extensive fund raising campaign advisory defibrillators were placed in each of the 500 or so emergency vehicles by the middle of 1990 and a sophisticated programme ("Heartstart Scotland") was initiated to follow and review the outcome of every ambulance resuscitation attempt.[3]

The ambulance service's contribution to the chain of survival

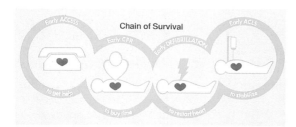

Chain of Survival

The concept of the chain of survival, with its four connecting links of early access to the emergency medical system, early cardiopulmonary resuscitation, early defibrillation, and early advanced life support,[4] together contributing to the optimum chance of survival after cardiac arrest, has been emphasised previously. The ambulance service is able to make useful contributions to each of these links in the chain.

Early access

The United Kingdom has had a dedicated emergency call number—999—to access the emergency services since 1937. Recently, attempts have been made to standardise an emergency call number—112—across Europe and a number of countries within the union respond to this instead of, or as well as, their national emergency number.

In the ambulance control a 999 call is taken by a control assistant working with control officers who, currently, detail the nearest available ambulance to the emergency in order of receipt of call. A number of systems are now available for prioritising the despatch of ambulances according to medically agreed criteria. This ensures that the most appropriate ambulance is despatched rapidly to calls of a life threatening nature. Speed of response is critical as survival after cardiorespiratory arrest falls exponentially with time.

In many services staff in ambulance control rooms are trained to provide emergency advice to the telephone caller including, when appropriate, instructions on how to perform cardiopulmonary resuscitation.

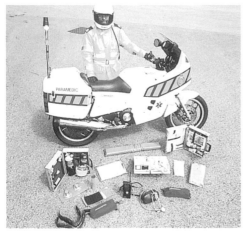

Motorcycles have been used to speed up the ambulance response in urban areas.

In cases of chest pain referred via the 999 system, calls for assistance receive a first priority response. The Heartstart Scotland scheme has shown that those patients who develop ventricular fibrillation *after* the arrival of the ambulance crew have a 50% chance of a long term survival. The ambulance controller should in addition ensure cases of suspected myocardial infarction are attended promptly by the general practitioner; a "dual response" should ensure that the patient is provided with effective analgesia, electocardiographic monitoring, defibrillation, and advanced life support when necessary. It will also allow prehospital thrombolysis when this could bring an important reduction in delay to treatment.

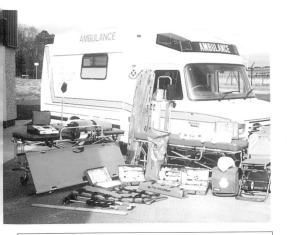

Early cardiopulmonary resuscitation

The benefits of early cardiopulmonary resuscitation have been well demonstrated, with survival from all forms of cardiac arrest almost doubling when cardiopulmonary resuscitation is undertaken. All emergency service staff should be trained in effective basic life support and their skills regularly refreshed and updated. In most parts of the United Kingdom ambulance service staff are also involved with training the general public in emergency life support, both at the instructor trainer level and, through organised community schemes, by direct contact with the public, schools, and local groups.

Early defibrillation

Every front line ambulance in the United Kingdom should now carry a defibrillator. Most often this is an advisory or automated external defibrillator, which can be operated by ambulance technicians; paramedics are trained and authorised to use manual defibrillators or, when available, automated external defibrillators with manual override devices.

The results of early defibrillation with automated external defibrillators operated by ambulance staff are encouraging. Between 1989 and 1993, 41 330 attempts at defibrillation were made by ambulance crews in the United Kingdom, with a return of spontaneous circulation achieved in 9104 (22%). In Scotland alone, where currently nearly 11 000 resuscitation attempts are logged on the database, 6332 patients have been defibrillated in five years with over 750 long term survivors; that is 200 survivors a year, an overall one year survival rate from out of hospital ventricular fibrillation of about 12%.

The introduction of automated external defibrillators has revolutionised defibrillation outside hospital. The sensitivity and specificity of these defibrillators is at least as good as for manual defibrillators used by paramedics; the time taken to defibrillate is less than with manual defibrillators.[5] They are supplied with high quality data recording, retrieval, and analysis systems and, most importantly, require only a few hours for operators to become competent in their use. The development of even simpler low cost units should extend the availability of defibrillation to any first responder, not just ambulance staff.

Equipment for front line ambulance

- Immediate response satchel (bag, valve, mask (adult and child); hand held suction; airways; laryngoscopy roll, endotracheal tubes; dressing pads; scissors)
- Portable oxygen therapy set
- Portable ventilator
- Defibrillator/monitor and accessories, pulse oximeter
- Sphygmomanometer and stethoscope
- Entonox
- Trolley cots, stretchers, poles, pillows, blankets
- Rigid collars
- Vacuum splints
- Spine immobiliser, long spine board
- Fracture splints
- Drugs packs, intravenous fluids, and cannulas
- Waste bins, sharps box
- Maternity pack
- Infectious diseases pack
- Hand lamp
- Rescue tools

Early advanced life support

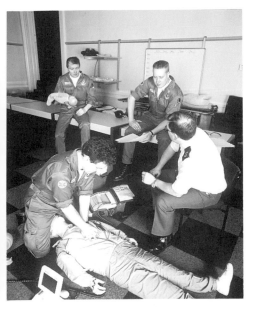

The NHS training directorate paramedic course adds to the already substantial basic training and experience given to ambulance technicians.[6] It emphasises the extended skills of venous cannulation, recording and interpreting electrocardiograms, intubation, infusion, defibrillation, and the use of selected drugs. The course is provided as an intensive nine week package, usually spread over several months. It covers the theoretical and practical knowledge needed for the extended care of emergency conditions in a minimum instruction period of 320 hours, four weeks of which is provided in hospital under the supervision of clinical tutors in cardiology, accident and emergency medicine, anaesthesia, and intensive care. A five day optional module covering training in emergency obstetric and neonatal resuscitation is also available.

Drugs sanctioned for use by trained ambulance staff

Drug	Route of administration
Oxygen	Inhalation/endotracheal
Entonox	Inhalation/endotracheal
Aspirin	Oral
Nitroglycerine	Sublingual
Adrenaline 1:10 000	Intravenous
Adrenaline 1:1 000	Intravenous; intramuscular
Lignocaine	Intravenous; endotracheal
Atropine	Intravenous; endotracheal
Diazepam	Intravenous; rectal
Salbutamol	Inhalation
Glucagon	Intravenous
Naloxone	Intravenous
Nalbuphine	Intravenous
Ergometrine	Intravenous
Sodium bicarbonate	Intravenous
Glucose infusion	Intravenous
Saline infusion	Intravenous
Ringer's lactate infusion	Intravenous
Polygeline infusion	Intravenous

In 1992 the Medicines Act was amended to permit ambulance paramedics to administer locally approved drugs from a range of prescription only medicines. The ability to provide early advanced life support other than defibrillation, for example advanced airway care, undoubtedly contributes to the overall success of ambulance based resuscitation.[7]

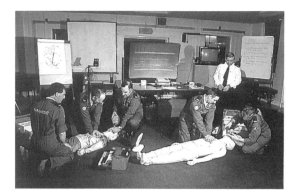

Retraining

Ambulance paramedics are subject to constant review and audit by local, medically constituted, paramedic steering committees. Paramedics must be refreshed in their skills annually and every three years attend a residential intensive revision course at an approved centre, with opportunities for further hospital placement if necessary.

The role of ambulance delivered advanced life support remains controversial and still has to be evaluated in comparison with prehospital advanced life support provided by medical practitioners. Much detailed study is required to assess the cost benefits of ambulance paramedics within the health service of the United Kingdom. The overwhelming impression is that they considerably enhance the professional image of the service and the quality of patient care.

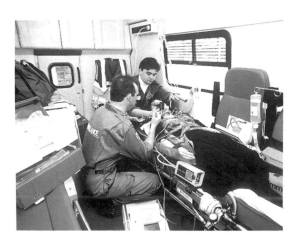

Coordination and audit

Local enthusiasm remains a cornerstone for developing resuscitation within the ambulance service. But a growing interest from the Department of Health and senior ambulance authorities is now leading to greater central encouragement and coordination.

The joint colleges ambulance liaison committee and the professional advisory group in Scotland includes participants from the colleges of physicians, surgeons, anaesthetists, general practitioners, and nurses and from the ambulance service. These bodies together provide a strong voice for prehospital care based on a sound medical and professional footing.

Outline syllabus for paramedic training

Theoretical knowledge

Basic anatomy and physiology:

- Respiratory system (especially mouth and larynx)
- Heart and circulation
- Central and autonomic nervous system

Presentation of common disorders:

- Respiratory obstruction, distress, or failure
- Presentations of ischaemic heart disease
- Differential diagnosis of chest pain
- Complications and management of acute myocardial infarction
- Acute abdominal emergencies
- Open and closed injury of chest and abdomen
- Limb fractures
- Head injury
- Fitting
- Burns
- Maxillofacial injuries
- Paediatric emergencies

Practical skills

Observing and assessing patient:

- Assessing the scene of the emergency
- Taking a brief medical history
- Observing general appearance, pulse, blood pressure (with sphygmomanometer), level of consciousness (with Glasgow scale)
- Undertaking systemic external examination for injury
- Recording and interpreting the electrocardiogram and rhythm monitor

Interventions

- Basic life support
- Defibrillation
- Intubation
- Venous cannulation and infusion
- Drug administration

A growing interest in extended ambulance training has brought increasing pressure for audit. The first national extended clinical audit was published by the NHS training authority in 1989. Since then annual returns have been collected on extended skills performed within each ambulance area. An audit subgroup of the joint colleges ambulance liaison committee coordinates collection of clinical data within the various ambulance services and oversees the processes of evaluating ambulance activity.

Benefits of resuscitation ambulances

The observed benefits of a resuscitation ambulance service include:
- Reduction in delay to hospital admission
- Successful cardiopulmonary resuscitation
- Increasing awareness of the need for rapid responses to emergencies
- Improved monitoring and support of the critically ill
- Improved standard of care for non-urgent cases.

The delay in time to hospital admission and the yearly number of successful resuscitations are the easiest benefits to quantify. Rates at well established centres vary between 20 and 100 successful resuscitations each year for populations of about 350 000; success means the subsequent discharge from hospital of an active and alert patient who would have stood no chance of survival without prehospital care. Techniques that provide comfort and prevent complications are less readily assessed but cannot be dismissed.

1 Partridge JF, Adgey AA, Geddes JS, Webb SW. *The acute coronary attack*. Tunbridge Wells: Pitman Medical, 1975.
2 Mackintosh A, Crabb ME, Granger R, Williams JH, Chamberlain DA. The Brighton resuscitation ambulances: review of 40 consecutive survivors of out of hospital cardiac arrest. *BMJ* 1978; i: 1115–8.
3 Cobbe SM, Redmond MJ, Watson JM, Hollingworth J, Carrington DJ. "Heartstart Scotland"–initial experience of a national scheme for out of hospital defibrillation. *BMJ* 1991, 302: 1517–20.
4 Cummins RO, Ornato JP, Thies WH, Pepe PE. Improving survival from sudden cardiac arrest: the "chain of survival" concept. *Circulation* 1991; **83**: 1832–47.
5 Sedgwick ML, Watson J, Dalziel K, Carrington DJ, Cobbe SM. Efficacy of out of hospital defibrillation by ambulance technicians using automatic external defibrillators. The Heartstart Scotland project. *Resuscitation* 1991; **24**: 73–87.
6 *Ambulance service paramedic training manual*. Bristol: National Health Service Training Directorate, 1991.
7 Lewis SJ, Homberg S, Quinn E, *et al*. Out of hospital resuscitation in East Sussex, 1981–1989. *Br Heart J* 1993; **70**: 568–73.

11 CARDIOPULMONARY RESUSCITATION AND THE GENERAL PRACTITIONER

Michael Colquhoun, Brian Steggles

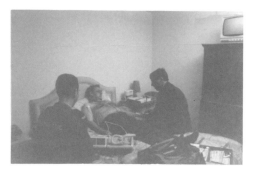

Myocardial infarction: a dual response by doctor and ambulance service.

Many more attempts are now being made in the community to resuscitate patients who suffer cardiopulmonary arrest. In many cases a general practitioner will contribute, either by initiating treatment or by working with the ambulance service. Sometimes a patient will experience a cardiac arrest actually in the presence of a general practitioner or the doctor will arrive shortly after the patient has collapsed; several studies have shown the effectiveness of resuscitation under these circumstances.

There are about 33 000 general practitioners in the United Kingdom working either alone or in group practices. Life threatening emergencies may present only rarely to an individual practitioner who, nevertheless, must be equipped to deal with the situation and must maintain his or her skills in resuscitation despite being expected to use them infrequently. There is, however, one condition, acute myocardial infarction, that is of particular importance to general practitioners because it is so common and because cardiac arrest occurs most commonly in the early stages—at the very time that the doctor is likely to be present.

Acute myocardial infarction

Myocardial infarction

Action by doctor

- Consider dual response
- Establish intravenous access
- Adequate pain relief to lessen risk of rhythm disturbance
- Use intravenous *not* intramuscular morphine or diamorphine with antiemetic
- Give aspirin
- Consider accompanying patient to hospital
- Consider thrombolytic therapy

All medical personnel who attend patients with myocardial infarction must be equipped to defibrillate.

It is estimated that about 300 000 people suffer a heart attack each year in the United Kingdom and about 125 000 of these patients die, most from ventricular fibrillation complicating the early stages.

In one series of 243 patients with cardiac arrest treated by general practitioners, acute myocardial infarction was the cause in nearly 70% and severe coronary artery disease without actual infarction accounted for most of the remainder. In only 12% of cases was cardiac arrest due to non-cardiac disease. Most of the patients with coronary disease collapsed in the presence of their doctor. The mechanism of cardiac arrest was ventricular fibrillation in nearly all cases, and two thirds of these patients reached hospital alive after defibrillation by the doctor, 60% being subsequently discharged home. Other studies have shown that about 5% of patients with acute infarction attended by a general practitioner experience a cardiac arrest in his or her presence.

These figures emphasise how important it is that general practitioners should be trained in resuscitation skills; it can no longer be considered sound practice knowingly to attend a case of acute myocardial infarction without being equipped to defibrillate. All front line ambulances in the United Kingdom now carry a defibrillator so if the general practitioner does not own one he or she should attend with the ambulance service. Such a dual response has several advantages in the management of acute myocardial infarction; the general practitioner will be aware of the patient's history and can provide diagnostic skills, administer opioid analgesics, and treat left ventricular failure and the ambulance service can provide the defibrillator and skilled help should cardiac arrest occur. Some practitioners will also administer thrombolytic treatment to patients with acute myocardial infarction and achieve a worthwhile saving in time compared with later administration in hospital.

Myocardial infarction and the practice team

Every practice should have a procedure for dealing with calls to potential cases of heart attack. Receptionists need to be aware of the importance of likely symptoms, particularly chest pain, and pass the call on to a doctor without delay. When the practice does not own a defibrillator the ambulance service should be summoned on a 999 basis to attend with the doctor. If the general practitioner cannot be contacted immediately or when there is likely to be a delay in attendance again the ambulance service should be summoned.

Cardiac arrest may occur on the surgery premises, perhaps when no doctor is immediately available. All reception and secretarial staff should therefore be competent in the techniques of basic life support with the use of a face mask or similar device, and the techniques should be practised regularly on a training manikin. Practice nurses must also be expert in performing basic life support, and when the practice owns a defibrillator they should be trained in its use. Such trained nurses can provide useful assistance on an emergency call.

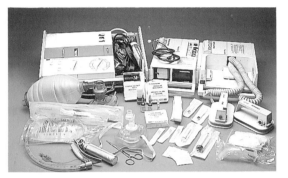

Equipment carried by GPs to patients with myocardial infarction.

Semiautomatic advisory defibrillators

The semiautomatic advisory defibrillator has been considered in detail in chapter 2. General practitioners need to be familiar with these machines and their method of operation so that they may work effectively with ambulance staff who are widely equipped with them. A practice contemplating the purchase of a defibrillator should consider the automated machine; skill in recognition of electrocardiographic rhythm is not required, and the automation of several stages in the process of defibrillation is a distinct advantage to the doctor who may well be working with very limited help.

Training the public

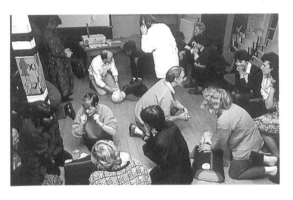

The influential 1987 report of the Royal College of Physicians, *Resuscitation from cardiopulmonary arrest: training and organisation*, recommended that general practitioners should "act as local co-ordinators for basic life support training and be encouraged to implement public education programmes in emergency aid for the area they serve." Recently there has been a lot of interest in training members of the lay public in the techniques of basic life support to increase the practice of cardiopulmonary resuscitation by bystanders. The promotion and coordination of such training is the purpose of *Heartstart UK* a national campaign promoted by the British Heart Foundation. General practitioners have already played an active part in several parts of the country, and it is to be hoped that this will increase in the future.

Immediate care schemes

In many parts of the United Kingdom specially trained and equipped general practitioners work closely with the emergency services to provide medical assistance in the resuscitation of victims of accidents and serious medical conditions. The emphasis is on team work; the doctor working closely with ambulance staff. Such schemes are coordinated by the British Association for Immediate Care (BASICS), which provides appropriate training courses and advice about equipment. The diploma in immediate medical care awarded by the Royal College of Surgeons of Edinburgh has established high standards for those who practise prehospital emergency care. For those who wish for extra knowledge and skills without aspiring to diploma level, a multidisciplinary prehospital emergency care course is run by the same Royal College in conjunction with BASICS.

Further reading

Weston CFM, Penny WJ, Julian DG on behalf of the British Heart Foundation Working Group. Guidelines for the early management of patients with myocardial infarction. *BMJ* 1994; **308**: 767–71.

Pai ER, Haites NE, Rawles JM, One thousand heart attacks in the Grampian; the place of cardiopulminary resuscitation in general practice. *BMJ* 1987; **29**: 352–4.

Colquhoun MC. The use of defibrillators by general practitioners. *BMJ* 1988; **297**: 336.

Colquhoun MC. Automated external defibrillation. *Br J Gen Pract* 1993; **43**: 95–6.

Rawlings DC. Study of the management of suspected cardiac infarction by British immediate care doctors. *BMJ* 1981; **282**: 1677–9.

Colquhoun MC, Julian DG. Treatable arrhythmias in cardiac arrests seen outside hospital. *Lancet* 1992; **339**: 1167.

12 NEAR DROWNING

Mark Harries

The clinical picture of near drowning is one of asphyxiation, often with pulmonary oedema due to water inhalation, in a profoundly cold subject. Complete recovery after 40 minutes' submersion in water has been documented. Unique clinical problems encountered in near drowning make its management different from all other emergencies in which cardiopulmonary arrest is a feature.

Incidence

Around 700 people drown each year in the United Kingdom, but the number of near drownings is not known. Male fatalities outnumber females by four to one, and in the age range 1 to 14 years only road traffic accidents and cancers account for more deaths. Two thirds die in inland waters and garden ponds and pools, where the opportunity to drown is greater than at the coast because of the lack of rescue services. Between a quarter and a half of drowned adults show evidence of excessive ingestion of alcohol.

Pathophysiology

Essential factors concerning the immersion incident	
Length of time submerged	Favourable outcome associated with submersion for less than 5 minutes
Quality of immediate resuscitation	Favourable outcome if heart beat can be restored at once
Temperature of the water	Favourable outcome associated with immersion in ice cold water (below 5°C) especially infant victims
Shallow water	Consider fracture/dislocation of cervical spine
A buoyancy aid being used by the casualty	Likely to be profoundly hypothermic. Victim may not have aspirated water. See postimmersion collapse
Nature of the water (fresh or salt)	Pulmonary oedema from fresh water inhalation more difficult to control. Risk of infection from river water high. Consider leptospirosis

Effects of cold

The thermal conductivity of water is greater than that of air so body cooling is much faster in water than in air at the same temperature. Sudden immersion of an unacclimatised subject in ice cold water results in reflex hyperventilation and tachycardia, often with supraventricular ectopic beats and hypertension, a response known as "cold shock"; drowning is likely to occur immediately unless a buoyancy aid is used. A clothed adult wearing a life jacket who enters water below 5°C can expect to lose consciousness within an hour of immersion. Cold also severely limits swimming ability because of loss of synchrony between stroke and breathing.

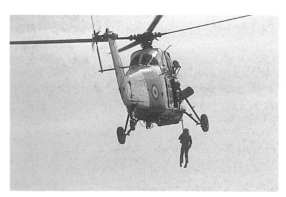

Circulatory collapse is believed to be the cause of death among those found unconscious in cold water wearing a life jacket but who die within minutes of being lifted out.

Collapse after immersion

Upright immersion in water with the head out results in greater than 30% increase in cardiac output because of the pressure exerted by the surrounding water. When the person leaves the water this support is suddenly removed. For normal people with intact homeostatic responses these changes are compensated for by baroreceptor reflexes which produce an increase in heart rate, cardiac output, and vascular smooth muscle tone. After prolonged immersion in cold water, however, these responses are compromised, resulting in circulatory collapse. This is believed to be the cause of death among those found conscious in cold water wearing life jackets but who die within minutes of rescue.

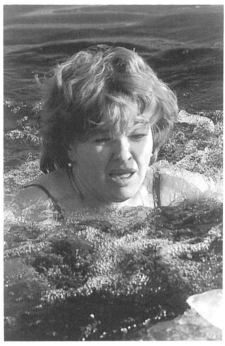

Sudden immersion in an unacclimatised subject in ice cold water results in reflux hyperventilation and tachycardia, often with supraventricular ectopic beats and hypertension, a condition known as cold shock; drowning is likely to occur immediately unless a buoyancy aid is used.

Infants show the apnoeic phase of the "diving response" when thrown into water, but this reflex tends to wane by the toddler stage. After infancy, submersion beyond the "breath hold breaking point" ends in involuntary gasps and aspiration of water. Postmortem measurements of lung weight, however, show that in up to 18% of drownings very little water is inhaled ("dry drowning").

Recovery from the asphyxia that follows a long period of submersion is more likely in circumstances that favour rapid cooling—for example, when a small child or infant is in ice cold water; several instances are recorded in which survival without brain damage has followed after up to 40 minutes under the water. In these circumstances circulatory arrest does not usually occur until after the head has become immersed so that cerebral perfusion continues during the cooling process.

Fluid and electrolyte effects

Fresh water washes out surfactant from the alveoli resulting in atelectasis and intrapulmonary shunting. On the other hand, salt water aspiration seems to be associated with very little alveolar-capillary damage.

Although red cell haemolysis does occur in fresh water drowning, changes in serum potassium concentrations are seldom important clinically; water intoxication leading to convulsions has been described in infants. Those electrolyte changes that occur in either form of drowning probably result from absorption of ingested fluid from the stomach. Raised serum sodium and magnesium concentrations may be found after immersion in sea water but seldom require treatment.

Emergency management

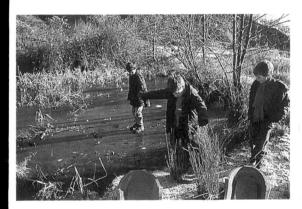

Swimmers recovered unconscious from shallow water should be assumed to have a fracture or dislocation of the cervical spine, particularly if there is injury to the face or head. Rupture of the liver or spleen has also been seen in those who have entered the water from a height.

The quality of the resuscitation procedure is the single most important factor in determining outcome. Cardiopulmonary resuscitation should be started immediately and should take precedence over all other considerations. It should not be abandoned while the subject remains cold. Regurgitation of gastric contents occurs in over half of near drowning casualties. The airway should therefore be secured with a tracheal tube at the earliest opportunity and oxygen given, preferably by using a rebreathing bag and reservoir to produce an inspired concentration near 100%.

In those who are profoundly cold the pulse may be slow and very difficult to feel. Great care is therefore needed when assessing the carotid pulse, and palpation for a period of at least 1 minute is recommended. An additional problem is that ventricular fibrillation may be precipitated by chest compression or by rough handling.

Management in hospital

Near drowning is a medical emergency. The casualty may present deeply unconscious with acidosis and profound hypothermia. Pulmonary oedema is an early complication. Cerebral oedema and septicaemia may develop later and are both life threatening.

Near drowning

Essential early measures

Tracheal intubation for unconscious victims	Secures the airway in the event of regurgitation
Electro-cardiogram	Pulseless patient may have bradyarrhythmias or ventricular fibrillation
Nasogastric tube	Decompresses the stomach thereby assisting ventilation. Reduces the risk of regurgitation
Rectal temperature	Use low reading thermometer. Insert the probe at least 10 cms
Arterial blood gases	Low PaO_2 breathing air is a marker for pulmonary oedema or atelectasis with shunting. A pH less than 7 associated with poor prognosis
Chest x ray examination	Shows aspirated fluid. Early indication of pulmonary oedema
Central venous line	Essential for monitoring level of positive end expiratory pressure respiration
Culture blood for both aerobic and anaerobic organisms	Septicaemia common. Consider "exotic" organisms. Brain abscess a late complication

Further measures

- Measure arterial gases
- In case of hypothermia raise core temperature above 28°C before defibrillation
- Consider plasma expanders and prophylactic antibiotics

Hypothermia

- Rewarm in bath water at 40°C
- Remove wet clothing if casualty can be sheltered
- Actively rewarm with extracorporeal bypass if necessary

Early measures

A detailed history of the accident will give an indication of the likely outcome. Those who are completely well may be discharged after a period of observation provided there are no lung crackles, the chest x ray picture shows no shadows, the respiratory rate is normal, there is no cough, and the arterial oxygen is normal with the subject breathing air. Anyone who has inhaled water is at risk of infection and should be followed up over the next day or so.

Unconscious patients require tracheal intubation and treatment with a high concentration of oxygen. Central venous access is required both to monitor pressure and to give fluids or drugs. An electrocardiogram may reveal bradyarrhythmias or ventricular fibrillation in those who at first seem to be pulseless.

Hypothermic subjects should be rewarmed while the rectal temperature is monitored with a low reading thermometer. The probe should be placed at least 10 cms beyond the anal sphincter to avoid erroneously low readings.

Blood should be drawn for both aerobic and anaerobic culture. Broad spectrum antibiotics effective against Gram negative organisms should be given.

Arterial blood gases

Arterial gases should be measured in all cases of near drowning. A pH of 7 or less is a poor prognostic sign. A low partial pressure of oxygen provides an early indication that water has been inhaled and identifies those at risk from pulmonary oedema. Modern analysers assume a normal body temperature of 37°C. Failure to allow for a low body temperature will result in a falsely high arterial oxygen reading.

The electrocardiogram

Nodal bradycardias are common, making the pulse difficult to find in some cases, but despite this there may be an adequate circulation.

Ventricular fibrillation associated with hypothermia responds poorly to direct current cardioversion. In this event the circulation must be supported by chest compression until the core temperature has been raised above 28°C, when defibrillation is more likely to be successful.

Venous pressure and intravenous drugs

The casualty's central venous pressure is often low initially, which is an indication for plasma expanders. Acidosis is usually self correcting once the circulation has been restored; administration of sodium bicarbonate is unnecessary. Systemic corticosteroids have not been shown to influence the course of pulmonary oedema and are not indicated. Antibiotics may be given prophylactically after a blood culture has been obtained.

Hypothermia

Conscious subjects may be hypothermic yet not shiver. Provided they are conscious enough to be cooperative, rewarming in bath water at 40°C is the treatment of choice. Those who are unconscious or uncooperative should be rewarmed passively by wrapping in thick woollen blankets or other insulating material. Wet clothing should be removed first provided this can be done while the casualty is sheltered from the elements.

A short lived fall in core temperature is commonly seen as rewarming commences and is known as the "after drop." It is caused by continued loss of heat through conduction from the core to the cooler peripheral tissues. It is not an adverse factor.

Active rewarming with extracorporeal bypass has been successful where passive measures have failed.

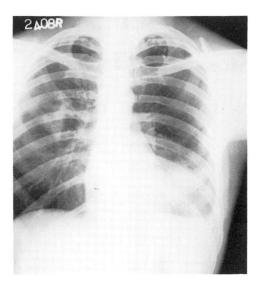

Shadowing in the left lower zone and right mid-zone represents aspirated water. The patient is at risk of developing the adult respiratory distress syndrome.

Pulmonary oedema

Pulmonary oedema occurs as a complication only in those who have inhaled water. Its onset is usually within four hours of aspiration, and an early sign is a falling arterial partial pressure of oxygen. An abnormal chest x ray picture or persisting crackles in the chest are also warning signs. Treatment is with positive end expiratory pressure (PEEP) respiration, which requires the patient to be intubated. The correct level of PEEP is that which maintains the arterial oxygen partial pressure above 10 kPa with a fractional inspired oxygen that should not exceed 0·6 in any 24 hour period.

Septicaemia

Lung infection is common after near drowning. Septicaemia and brain abscesses have also been reported suggesting arterial embolisation of infected material, possibly the result of pulmonary barotrauma. Infection may be overwhelming, and death has been caused by opportunistic organisms such as *Aspergillus fumigatus*. Leptospirosis is another hazard that is well recognised in sportsmen using inland waters. Victims of immersion should be warned that a fever developing within a few days of the accident should be taken seriously, and they should be offered follow up with a chest x ray examination.

13 AIDS, HEPATITIS, AND RESUSCITATION

David A Zideman

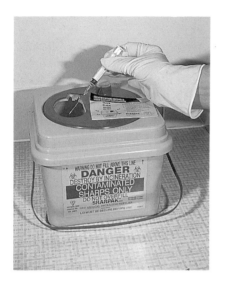

In cardiopulmonary resuscitation there is no reason to delay basic life support (airway, breathing, and circulation) until the possible infective state of the patient has been established. A great deal has been written by knowledgeable authors and by others about the risk of contact of health care workers, resuscitators, first aiders, and the general public with blood or body fluids of patients being resuscitated who are considered to be possible carriers of HIV or hepatitis B virus. In response to ill founded concern prompted by the ill informed and the media, concerning the perceived risks of salivary exposure many "alternative methods" have been recommended.

Guidelines

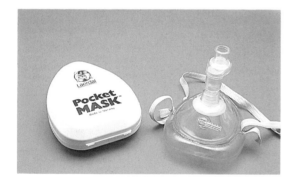

The Laerdal pocket mask incorporating a disposable filter and one way valve.

A report from the Centers for Disease Control updated previous advice on universal precautions against parenteral, mucous membrane, or non-intact skin exposures to HIV or hepatitis B virus.[1] It emphasised the fact that blood is the single most important source of these viruses and applied its recommendations for universal precaution to semen, vaginal secretions, and cerebrospinal, synovial, pleural, peritoneal, pericardial, and amniotic fluid and to any body fluid containing visible blood. Body fluids to which these universal precautions do not apply include sputum, nasal secretions, faeces, sweat, tears, urine, and vomit unless they contain visible blood. A series of epidemiological studies of the non-sexual contacts of patients with HIV suggested that the possibility of salivary transmission of HIV is remote,[2-6] and a further study showed that hepatitis B was not transmitted from resuscitation manikins.[7]

Protective airway devices

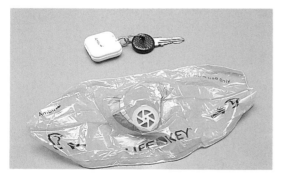

The Ambu Lifekey contains a barrier device in a keyring.

Despite the above, some health care workers and members of the general public may feel the need for some interpositional airway device, for example in accident departments when the saliva of trauma victims may be contaminated with blood. Before selecting such a device the user must be satisfied that it will function effectively in its resuscitation and protective roles and must be properly trained in its use, regularly tested in its use, properly informed about its cleaning, sterilisation, and disposal, and must be assured of its immediate availablity at times of cardiopulmonary resuscitation.

Needlestick injuries

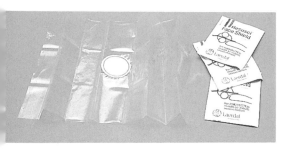

The Laerdal Faceshield: a plastic sheet incorporating a filter.

Resuscitation is an emergency procedure that does include, in its advanced stages, invasive techniques. Special care must be taken to ensure that, in the hustle and bustle of resuscitation, members of the resuscitation team are not accidentally contaminated with possibly infected material and are carefully guarded against needlestick and "sharp" injuries. Sharp disposal boxes should be part of resuscitation equipment. The decision about how many more of the recommended universal precautions should be applied should be based on the prevalence of HIV and hepatitis B virus in the locality.

Training manikins

Practice in resuscitation techniques is an essential part of establishing an effective resuscitation service. Resuscitation training manikins have not been shown to be sources of virus infection. Nevertheless, sensible precautions must be taken to minimise potential cross infection, and the manikins must be formally disinfected after each use according to the manufacturers' recommendations.

Conclusion

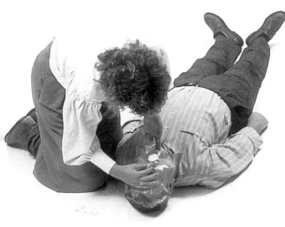

Use of a face shield during mouth to mouth ventilation.

Interpositional airway adjuncts are not essential for performing mouth to mouth resuscitation but, if a patient's oral cavity or saliva is contaminated with visible blood, the use of an adjunct can reassure the rescuer. Starting mouth to mouth respiration must not be delayed until such an airway adjunct is provided.

1 Centers for Disease Control. Update: universal precautions for prevention of transmission of human immunodeficiency virus, hepatitis B virus and other blood-borne pathogens in health care settings. *MMWR* 1988; **37**: 377–88.
2 Centers for Disease Control. Update: acquired immunodeficiency syndrome and human immunodeficiency virus infection among health care workers. *MMWR* 1988; **37**: 229–34, 239.
3 Friedland GH, Saltzman BR, Rogers MF, *et al.* Lack of transmission of HTLV-III/LAV infection to household contacts of patients with AIDS or AIDS related complex with oral candidiasis. *N Engl J Med* 1986; **314**: 344–9.
4 Jason JM, McDougal JS, Dixon G, *et al.* HTLV III-LAV antibody and immune status of household contacts and sexual partners of persons with hemophilia. *JAMA* 1986; **255**: 212–5.
5 Curran JW, Jaffe HW, Hardy AM, *et al.* Epidemiology of HIV infection and AIDS in the United States. *Science* 1988; **239**: 610–6.
6 Lifson AR. Do alternative modes for transmission of human immunodeficiency virus exist? A review. *JAMA* 1988; **259**: 1353–6.
7 Glaser JB, Nadler JP. Hepatitis B virus in a cardiopulmonary resuscitation training course: risk of transmission from a surface antigen-positive participant. *Arch Intern Med* 1985; **145**: 1653–5.

14 TRAINING IN RESUSCITATION TECHNIQUES

Michael Colquhoun, Andrew H Swain, Anthony J Handley

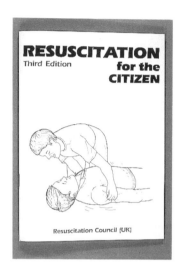

Several developments in the teaching of both basic and advanced life support have occurred in the United Kingdom in recent years. The increased capability of the ambulance service to resuscitate victims of out of hospital cardiac arrest has focused attention on the need to train members of the public in basic life support skills. If cardiopulmonary resuscitation is performed by bystanders who witness cardiac arrest, subsequent efforts by the emergency service will be successful more often.

Improved training for hospital staff has been achieved with the appointment of resuscitation training officers in many health districts throughout the country. The resuscitation training officer coordinates training in both basic and advanced life support, providing tuition to employees appropriate to their requirements. An important advance in the teaching of advanced skills has been the development of the advanced life support course pioneered in the United Kingdom by the Resuscitation Council (UK).

Training the public

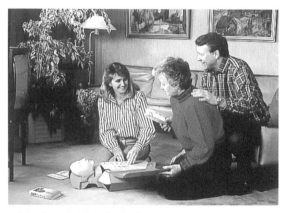

The Laerdal Family Trainer is an inexpensive manikin that enables practice in basic life support.

Several studies from North America and Europe have shown the value of basic life support initiated by bystanders before the arrival of the emergency medical services. One recent report from Scotland has confirmed that these benefits are also achievable with the emergency systems and ambulance response times that exist in the British Isles.

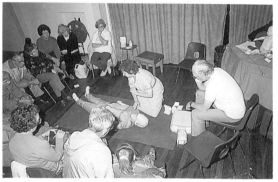

Citizen cardiopulmonary resuscitation class.

Basic life support is effective because it delays the degeneration of ventricular fibrillation into terminal asystole; the patient is more likely to be in ventricular fibrillation when the ambulance arrives and so respond to defibrillation. Research in the United States, most notably from Seattle and King County in Washington State, has shown that basic life support must be initiated within four minutes of the patient's collapse to give the best chance of successful resuscitation. In some American cities, for example Milwaukee, the emergency services are themselves able to attend patients within this time limit; this would be very unusual in the British Isles.

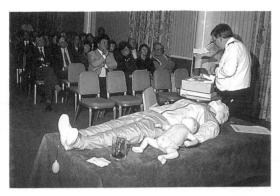

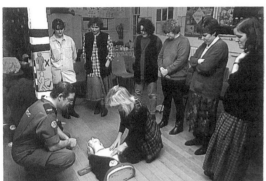

Citizen cardiopulmonary resuscitation class.

Campaigns to teach basic life support to members of the public gained momentum in the early 1990s with the move to equip every front line ambulance with a defibrillator. In the United Kingdom, training for basic life support is provided by the voluntary aid societies and the Royal Life Saving Society UK, but it is not routinely taught in schools. Pioneering schemes to teach the public have been instigated by enthusiasts in some areas of the country—for example, Brighton (Heart Guard), Malvern (Heartstart), and the City of London (Bart's City Life Saver).

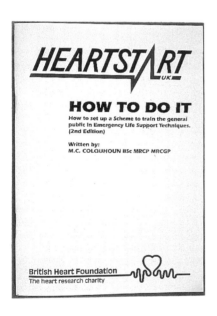

More recently the British Heart Foundation has taken a lead in promoting such schemes through the Heartstart UK initiative, acting in a facilitatory role to provide practical help through their professional coordinators. They have also produced a range of teaching aids and support material. As a result of the Heartstart UK initiative several schemes have been established to teach basic life support in a single session of about two hours. Instruction on the treatment of choking and use of the recovery position is included. The basic syllabus is covered in the booklet *Resuscitation for the citizen* published by the Resuscitation Council (UK), and detailed information about running such schemes is contained in *Heartstart – how to do it* published by the British Heart Foundation. Trainers from the statutory ambulance services and the voluntary first aid and lifesaving societies have undertaken most training in the schemes so far established. Practising the techniques on training manikins is an essential part of these classes and reinforces the theoretical instruction that is provided.

Schools

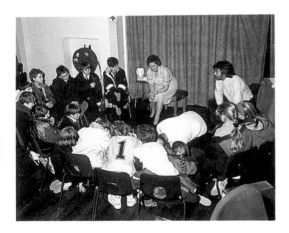

The teaching of first aid is not universal in British schools nor is a knowledge of first aid required of every teacher. The subject is included within the National Curriculum in England and Wales but is not compulsory at the present time. In contrast, basic life support skills have been taught regularly at school in some European countries, most notably Norway, for the past 30 years, and successful application of the techniques has been reported.

Advanced life support courses

The first formal training in the management of cardiopulmonary arrest was introduced by the American Heart Association in 1975. The course in advanced cardiac life support combines both tuition and testing according to the guidelines of the American Heart Association.

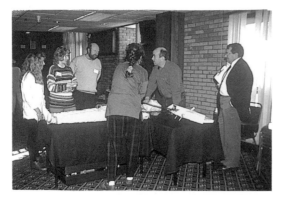

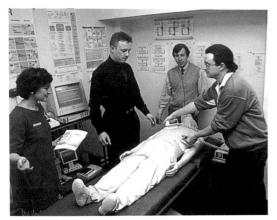

Simulated cardiac arrest practice on an advanced life support course.

In the United Kingdom a series of papers published between 1984 and 1987 reported serious deficiencies in the ability of nurses and junior hospital doctors to perform both basic and advanced life support. The 1987 Royal College of Physicians report *Resuscitation from cardiopulmonary arrest: training and organisation* recommended that regular training in the management of cardiopulmonary arrest should be undertaken by all doctors, medical students, nurses, dental practitioners, and paramedical staff. The first advanced life support course, modelled on the American course but following the guidelines of the Resuscitation Council (UK), was held at St Bartholomew's Hospital, London, in 1987. Similar courses took place in other areas of the country, and in 1990 the Resuscitation Council (UK) formed a multidisciplinary body to promote the development of a national course. This became available in 1993 and consists of a course programme, manual, and a standardised set of slides for use by lecturers.

The object of the advanced life support course is to teach both the theory and practical skills required to manage cardiopulmonary arrest in adults until the patient is able to enter the intensive care unit or has died. The course is appropriate for medical, nursing, and paramedical staff. A uniform approach is adopted so that participants are trained to the same standard whatever their grade and wherever the course is held. The protocols used in the management of the three forms of cardiac arrest (ventricular fibrillation, asystole, and electromechanical dissociation) are those of the European Resuscitation Council.

The course lasts a minimum of two days and is very intensive. The manual is designed for reading before the course and is sent to all participants one month in advance together with a multiple choice question paper.

Competence in basic life support is essential and participants must pass a test, similar to that required for membership of the Royal College of General Practitioners, on the first day of the course. The emphasis throughout is on practical skills, formal lectures occupying less than half of the programme.

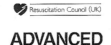

ADVANCED LIFE SUPPORT MANUAL

2nd EDITION – 1994

Practical skill stations cover the following topics: basic life support, basic and advanced airway management, recognition of arrhythmias, defibrillation with both manual and semiautomatic defibrillators, and the use of drugs. The team approach to cardiac arrest management is learnt in the environment of a simulated cardiac arrest. This poses the greatest challenge to course participants; the scenarios are designed to be as realistic as possible with modern training manikins and resuscitation equipment. The simulated cardiac arrest develops team leadership and integrates the theoretical and practical teaching.

Useful addresses

The British Heart Foundation
14 Fitzhardinge Street
London W1H 4DH

The Resuscitation Council (UK)
9 Fitzroy Square
London W1P 5AH

The British Red Cross Society
9 Grosvenor Crescent
London SW1X 7EJ

The Royal Life Saving Society UK
Mountbatten House
Studley
Warwickshire B80 7NN

St Andrew's Ambulance Association
St Andrew's House
48 Milton Street
Glasgow G4 0HR

St John Ambulance
1 Grosvenor Crescent
London SW1X 7EF

In the final session of the course candidates are tested by means of a multiple choice question paper and an arrhythmia recognition test together with assessment of their skill at airway control, defibrillation, and the management of simulated cardiac arrest. Uniform criteria are used for the assessments to ensure each course reaches the same national standard. Successful candidates receive a Resuscitation Council (UK) advanced life support certificate valid for three years; criteria for reaccreditation have also been agreed. Course participants who show outstanding ability are invited to attend a two day instructor course, which is supervised by an educationalist and focuses on teaching techniques such as lecturing and management of skill stations.

Careful monitoring and supervision is necessary to ensure the quality and standardisation of all advanced life support courses. To this end each course has to be registered, and the course programme and faculty of teachers must be approved by the Resuscitation Council (UK). It is hoped that the course will become established throughout the country, extend into the undergraduate curriculum, and be compatible with similar initiatives in Europe. In this way disorganised and fraught attempts at cardiopulmonary resuscitation will become a thing of the past.

"Resuscitation for the Citizen" (3rd edition) is obtainable from The Resuscitation Council (UK).

15 TRAINING AND RETENTION OF SKILLS

Geralyn Wynne

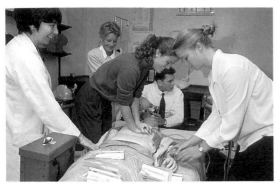

Simulated cardiac arrest training: medical students.

Resuscitation involves skills that are essentially practical, and students need practical training to acquire them. Life threatening events rarely occur at a time or place where teaching is possible so training has to be given in simulated situations. This has been made possible by the development of various training manikins and teaching aids.

Several surveys have highlighted the inability of house officers and nurses to perform cardiopulmonary resuscitation and have shown an urgent need for a review of training methods. Formal training should begin in medical and nursing school and be repeated regularly. During subsequent revision sessions no assumptions should be made about previous knowledge or skill.

Levels of training

The Royal College of Physicians' 1987 report *Resuscitation from cardiopulmonary arrest: training and organisation*[1] suggested that resuscitation skills should be divided into separate levels of attainment:

Basic life support – This comprises initial assessment of a casualty, maintenance of the airway, expired air ventilation, and support of the circulation by chest compression. Basic life support should be taught to all nurses, physiotherapists, radiographers, preclinical medical students, and other staff who are in contact with patients. The general public also should be trained in these skills.

Basic life support with airway adjuncts – The use of simple mechanical airways and devices such as the facemask should be taught to general medical practitioners, qualified nursing staff, ambulance technicians, and clinical medical students.

Basic life support with airway adjuncts plus defibrillation – The use of defibrillators (semiautomatic or manual) should be taught to hospital medical staff (including house officers and locum hospital doctors), specially trained nursing staff (working in hospital areas such as coronary care units, intensive treatment units, and accident and emergency departments), and ambulance staff. Training should also be offered to general practitioners.

Advanced life support (ALS) – Advanced life support should be taught to medical and nursing staff who are, or who may be, members of a hospital resuscitation team, to ambulance paramedics, and to those general practitioners who wish to acquire these special skills.

Nurse receiving instruction in defibrillation.

Retention of skill

Since the American Heart Association published its original resuscitation standards in 1974[2] investigators in the United States have studied the question of how students learn and how they retain resuscitation skills.

Performance deteriorates with time; this can be shown even six weeks after training and severe loss of skill occurs after about 12 months, when 20% or fewer can still perform basic life support proficiently. Decline in resuscitation skills is greater than for other first aid skills such as applying traction, splinting, or bandaging.

A British study evaluated the ability of occupational first aiders to carry out cardiopulmonary resuscitation at varying times up to three years after training; only 12% of those tested would have been capable of performing effective cardiopulmonary resuscitation. The study also showed that there was a rapid and linear decay in resuscitation skills

> **Skills not regularly practised are not retained**

over time, with fewer than 20% of the subjects achieving a score of 75% six months after training.[3]

The underlying message is clear: skills that are not regularly practised are not retained. A study conducted in the Netherlands suggested that "refresher training" should take place every six months to maintain proficiency in basic life support.[4]

The attainment and subsequent retention of skills depends on the course content and the time devoted to manikin practise. Unfortunately many cardiopulmonary resuscitation programmes do not give trainees the opportunity to attain a high level of performance; if the initial level of skill is low, retention will be poorer. For example, trainees who complete eight hours of instruction show less deterioration in skill than those who complete a four hour course; after one year, however, even their skills are below standard.

Do people who perform "poorly" in studies of skill retention lack the ability to provide effective cardiopulmonary resuscitation on humans? Some studies have shown that poor technique is related to a poor outcome for the victim, although others have failed to identify any relation between technique and survival.

In some cases, the reason for poor performance seems to be the reluctance of rescuers to undertake expired air ventilation. The acceptability of this technique of ventilation was surveyed among 70 medical and nursing staff. Sixty four of those questioned were not prepared to ventilate "dirty patients" (those who had vomited, had dirty sputum, or were infected) with the mouth to mouth technique, and 27 would not use mouth to mask ventilation.[5] Oral adjuncts, such as the pocket face mask, which avoid the need for direct contact with patients need to be introduced to overcome these objections.

> Experience gained at cardiac arrests is not a substitute for formal practical training

Advanced life support (see chapters 2, 3, 4, and 5)

The purpose of a course in advanced life support is to provide doctors, nurses, medical students, paramedics, and allied health care staff with adequate knowledge and practical skills to give definitive treatment to patients who suffer cardiopulmonary arrest. It should include simulated cardiac arrests at which students integrate their knowledge and skills by recognising arrhythmias, performing defibrillation, practising intravenous cannulation and tracheal intubation, managing the airway, and giving drug treatment, thereby acting as members of a coordinated resuscitation team.

Evaluation of the training afforded by simulated cardiac arrest scenarios has shown improvement in performance during real resuscitation attempts. The observed improvements are greater efficiency and credibility, quicker decision making, improved communication skills, and reduction in anxiety and confusion.

Reinforcement and continuing medical education may enhance retention of knowledge but may not maintain psychomotor skills. Yearly recertification in advanced life support should be considered, and frequent simulated practice sessions should be encouraged for doctors and nurses.

One factor which may adversely affect the acquisition of both basic and advanced resuscitation skills is overconfidence. About 78% of medical students and residents questioned felt confident in their ability to perform basic resuscitation but only 2·9% were able to give a correct demonstration. Trained nurses of sister/charge nurse grade felt considerably more confident than staff nurses at performing basic resuscitation, but they were no more competent when tested. This large discrepancy between imagined and actual ability means that many professional people are unaware of their need for additional training.

The Resuscitation Council (UK) has attempted to deal with the problem of poor acquisition and retention of skills by producing an advanced life support course based upon European standards and guidelines (see chapter 14).

Feedback has been shown to be an important component of teaching programmes as it highlights both proficiencies and deficiencies in skills thus encouraging students to practise further to improve their performance. Feedback of performance of basic resuscitation skills can be given to the student by visual signals or a paper recording from the manikin or by the instructor.

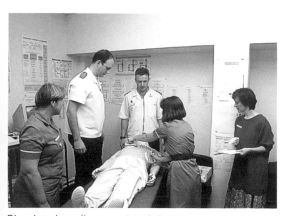

Simulated cardiac arrest training.

Quality of trainers

It is usually assumed that teachers of resuscitation are competent at the technique themselves; however, this is seldom evaluated. Studies of the performance of trainers in America and the United Kingdom have found deviations from the standard training programme and an inability of the instructors themselves to perform basic life support. These factors may be another reason for poor acquisition and retention of resuscitation skills.

Suggested teaching technique

A four step technique can be valuable in the teaching of psychomotor skills:

- The instructor performs a silent run through of the skill
- The instructor repeats the demonstration with a commentary
- The student gives a commentory as the instructor demonstrates
- The student demonstrates the skill with commentary.

This technique provides good feedback to the students, but it is important to maintain continuity and a smooth transition from one phase to the next. The groups should be small, ideally four to six people, to allow maximum time for the acquisition of skills and to allow feedback to the student about their performance.

> **Confidence is not related to competence**

1 Royal College of Physicians. Resuscitation from cardiopulmonary arrest: training and organisation. *J R Coll Physicians Lond* 1987; **21**: 1–8.
2 American Heart Association. Standards and guidelines for cardiopulmonary resuscitation and emergency cardiac care. *JAMA* 1974; **227**: 833–68.
3 McKenna SP, Glendon AI. Occupational first aid training. Decay in CPR skills. *Journal of Occupational Psychology* 1985; **58**: 109–17.
4 Benden HJJM, Williams FF, Hendrick JMA, *et al*. How frequently should basic cardiopulmonary resuscitation training be repeated to maintain adequate skills. *BMJ* 1993; **306**: 1576–7.
5 Lawrence PJ, Sivaneswaran N. Ventilation during CPR, which method? *Anaesthetics and Intensive Care* 1985; **13**: 201.

16 TRAINING MANIKINS

Michael Colquhoun, R S Simons

Resuscitation skills that can be practiced on manikins

Basic life support
- Manual airway control ± simple airway adjuncts
- Pulse detection
- Expired air ventilation (mouth to mouth or mouth to mask)
- Chest compression
- Treatment of choking
- The recovery position

Advanced techniques
- Precordial thump
- Airway adjuncts
- Oropharyngeal suction
- Ventilation devices—for example, bag/valve/mask
- Tracheal intubation
- Interpretation of electrocardiographic arrhythmia
- Defibrillation and cardioversion
- Intravenous and intraosseous access (± administration of drugs)

Related skills
- Management of haemorrhage, fractures, and other trauma
- Treatment of pneumothorax
- Nursing care skills
- Rescue and transport

Both theoretical and practical skills are required to learn cardiopulmonary resuscitation techniques. Whereas theoretical skills can be learnt in the classroom from written material or from computer programs, the acquisition of practical skills requires the use of training manikins. Suitable manikins have been developed since the original description of expired air ventilation and external cardiac compression because of the realisation that it is impracticable as well as potentially dangerous to practice these procedures on human volunteers. Manikins are available for the practice of almost all the techniques in cardiopulmonary resuscitation.

Adult and paediatric manikins are available from several manufacturers worldwide; this chapter concentrates on those generally available in the United Kingdom.

Manikin selection – general principles

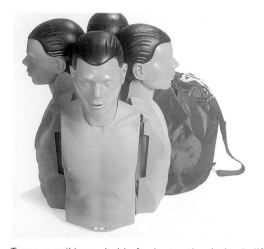

Torso manikins suitable for instruction in basic life support.

Training requirements

Choice of manikin will obviously depend on the skill of the class under instruction; the requirements of a class to teach cardiopulmonary resuscitation to lay people for example will be quite different from those of a class for professional hospital staff. With all manikins, realistic appearance and accurate anatomical landmarks are essential. The response of the manikin to any attempted resuscitation manoeuvre should be realistic and occur only when it is performed correctly – for example, many manikins for teaching basic life support will usually allow chest expansion only when the airway is patent.

Many manikins are available as torso models, although limbs are often available as an optional extra. Torso models are cheaper than a whole body manikin, and the reduced size and weight make storage and transport easier; they are of course less lifelike.

Training manikins

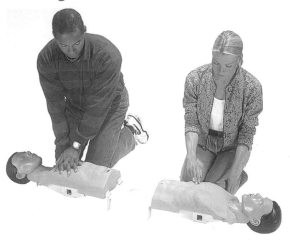

Simple torso manikins (Ambu) suitable for instruction in basic life support.

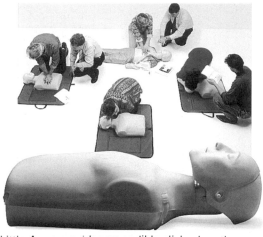

Little Anne provides an audible click when the correct depth of chest compression is achieved.

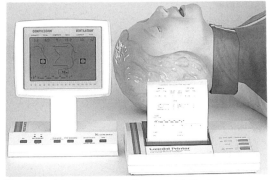

The Laerdal skill meter offers sophisticated assessment of students' performance.

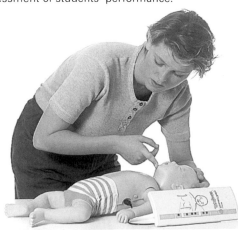

Lifelike infant resuscitation can be practised using Resusci Baby, which incorporates sensors and flashing indicators to provide feedback to student and instructor.

Visual display and recording

Manikins differ in the amount of feedback they give to both student and instructor and in their ability to provide details about performance. Models vary greatly in sophistication, but most provide some qualitative indication that technique is adequate, such as audible clicks when the depth of chest compression is correct. Some manikins incorporate sensors that recognise a correct hand position, and the rescuer's attempts at shaking, opening the airway, and palpation of a pulse. The depths of ventilation and chest compression may also be recorded. An objective assessment of performance may be communicated to the student or instructor by means of flashing lights, meters, audible signals, or graphical display on a screen. A permanent record may be obtained for subsequent study or certification.

Manikins that interface with computers will measure performance for a set period and compare adequacy of technique against established standards such as those of the European Resuscitation Council or the American Heart Association. A score of the number of correct manoeuvres may form the basis of a test of competence; however, the software algorithms in some assessment programs are very strict, and only minimal deviation from these standards is tolerated. A minimum score of 70% correct cardiac compressions and ventilations represents effective life support. This score on a Skillmeter Resusci Anne mannikin is acceptable to the Royal College of General Practitioners of the United Kingdom for the award of a resuscitation certificate.

Maintenance and repair

Manikins should be easy to clean. The "skin" should not be permanently marked by lipstick or pens or allowed to become stained with extensive use. Proprietary cleaning fluids, many based on alcohol, are available, and the manufacturer's instructions should be followed in all cases. Many currently available manikins have replacements available for those components subject to extensive wear and tear. This is particularly true for the face skin, which bears the brunt of damage and where discoloration or wear will make the manikin aesthetically unattractive.

Manikins are bulky and require adequate space for both maintenance and storage. A carrying case (preferably rigid and fitted with castors for heavier manikins) is essential for safe storage and transport.

Cross infection and safety

To minimise the risks of infection occurring during the conduct of simulated mouth to mouth ventilation the numbers of students using each manikin should be kept low and careful attention should be paid to hygiene (handwashing etc). Students should be free of communicable infection, particularly of the face, mouth, or respiratory tract. Faceshields or other barrier devices (see chapter 13) should be used when appropriate. Manikins should be disinfected during and after each training session; preparations incorporating 70% alcohol and chlorhexidine are often used. Hypochlorite solutions containing 500 ppm chlorine (prepared by adding 20 ml of domestic bleach to one litre of water) are effective but unpleasant to use. They are best reserved for the thorough cleaning of manikins between classes. Molded hair has now replaced stranded or artificial hair and is much easier to keep clean.

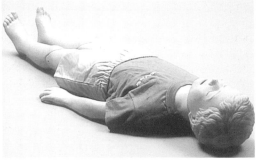

Resusci Junior (Laerdal) simulates a five year old child and can also be used for water rescue techniques.

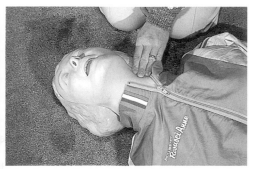

Ambu manikin.

Many modern manikins feature a disposable lower airway consisting of plastic lungs and connecting tubes. Expired air passes through a non-return valve to the side of the manikin during expiration. All disposable parts should be replaced in accordance with the maker's recommendations. Other manikins use a clean mouthpiece and disposable plastic bag insert for each student. An individual head bag ensures that no contact can be made with other students' breath; the exhalation of the same air that the student has used to inflate the manikin provides a realistic simulation of the expiratory phase of ventilation as the student can hear and feel breath returning through the upper airway. After each training session the head bag is discarded and the face piece is disinfected.

Cost

Costs will depend on the skills to be practiced and the number of manikins required for a class. Increasingly sophisticated skills, monitoring, recording, and reporting facilities increase cost further. Any budget should include an allowance for cleaning, disposables, and replacements.

Manikin requirements for basic life support

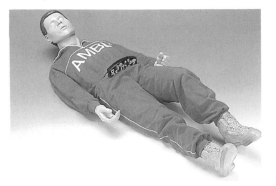

Palpation of the pulse on a Skillmeter Resusci Anne (Laerdal).

Airway

The facility to open the airway by tilting the neck or lifting the jaw, or both, is a feature of practically all manikins currently available. Modern manikins cannot be ventilated unless the appropriate steps to secure a patent airway have been taken.

Regrettably, some manikins require excessive neck extension to secure airway patency; such action would be quite inappropriate in the presence of an unstable injury to the cervical spine.

Back blows and abdominal thrusts used to treat the choking casualty can be practiced convincingly only on a manikin made specially for the purpose; some degree of simulation, however, is possible with most manikins.

Breathing

Most currently available manikins offer realistic simulation of chest wall compliance and resistance to expired air ventilation. In some manikins attempts to inflate the chest when the airway is inadequately opened or the use of excessive pressure will result in distension of the "stomach." Some advanced manikins feature a stomach bag that may be emptied by the instructor under appropriate circumstances and used to simulate regurgitation into the casualty's mouth.

Mouth to nose ventilation is difficult to perform on some manikins because the nose is small, too soft, too hard, or has inadequate nostrils. Access for nasal catheters and airways is impracticable on most manikins for this reason.

The design of most basic manikins does not readily permit the use of simple airway adjuncts (for example, the Guedel airway) as space in the oropharynx and hypopharynx is limited; special airway trainers are more suitable for this purpose. The quality of ventilation with a facemask depends on the seal between the mask and face of the manikin; a mask with an inflatable cuff will provide better contact and seal. Similar considerations apply when a bag valve mask device is used. The rather rigid and inflexible face of most manikins dictates that a firm one handed grip is required to prevent air leaks; as in real life a two handed grip may be required on such occasions.

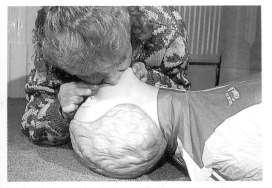

Performing expired air ventilation on a training manikin.

Training manikins

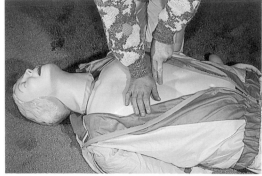

Identifying the correct position for chest compression.

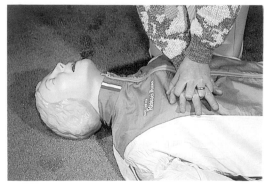

Performing chest compression on a training manikin.

Circulation

Several manikins have a palpable pulse that is simulated either electronically or manually by squeezing an air bulb attached to the manikin by plastic tubing. In adult manikins the carotid pulse is used whereas in infant or baby manikins the brachial artery is palpated.

Chest compression should be practiced on manikins with appropriate chest wall compliance and recoil. Many manikins have some form of indication that the depth of compression is adequate, and some will monitor hand position. Few if any manikins allow carotid pulsation to be activated by rescuer chest compression.

The recovery position

Adoption of the recovery position is impracticable with manikins lacking flexible bodies and jointed limbs; in most cases a human volunteer is more practicable and realistic.

Manikin requirement for advanced life support

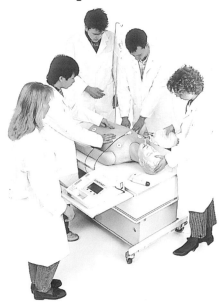

Group instruction in management of cardiac arrest employing a training manikin (Laerdal).

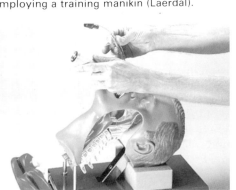

Manikin for practising tracheal intubation (Ambu).

A few advanced manikins allow tasks to be undertaken concurrently (for example, basic life support, electrocardiographic monitoring, defibrillation, tracheal intubation, and intravenous cannulation). Without such advanced equipment it used to be necessary to arrange several different manikins in the training room or incorporate elements of several models to construct a special manikin. The team management of cardiac arrest can now be practiced in an interactive fashion and some models permit the instructor to alter conditions and present an evolving scenario. Documentation of events during the simulated resuscitation attempt and the response to therapeutic interventions is possible, and a detailed report subsequently allows the supervisor to assess the performance of the team collectively and individually. Imaginative changes of attire, location, and access are also possible to present the team with training in different environments; this is relevant for training in both cardiac and trauma life support.

Some manikins feature optional additional extras that allow the simulation of a variety of injuries (for example, burns, lacerations, and fractures). Other models permit the procedures of transtracheal jet ventilation, cricothyrotomy, pericardiocentesis, surgical venous access, and tube thoracostomy. Features such as these have proved invaluable to those concerned with trauma care.

Tracheal intubation

The technique of tracheal intubation is difficult to acquire; it requires training, practice, and continuous experience. Specially designed manikins are available for the purpose but are costly, difficult to manufacture, and expensive to maintain. Manikins dedicated to the teaching of airway management feature a head and neck containing an accurate simulation of the anatomy of the oropharynx and larynx.

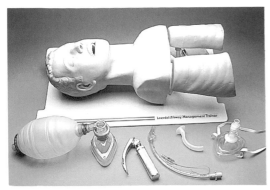

Airway management trainer (Laerdal) allows ventilation of the manikin with a range of airway adjuncts including tracheal intubation.

These models are usually mounted on a rigid baseboard that ensures stability while the head and neck are manoeuvred. The range of airway adjuncts that may be used include oropharyngeal airways, the laryngeal mask airway, bag valve mask devices, and tubes. The nasopharynx is usually accurately represented, allowing nasal intubation and the use of nasopharyngeal airways. Oropharyngeal suction may also be practised. One model currently available features a cutaway of the left side of the face and neck that improves visualisation of technique being used, although not bag mask valve ventilation. Infant and neonatal models are available.

Careful choice of a robust airway management trainer is recommended, and lubricant spray should always be used. Damage to the mouth, tongue, epiglottis, and larynx is common, and repair or replacement of these parts should be easy and relatively inexpensive.

Electrocardiographic monitoring and rhythm recognition

The ability to monitor and interpret the cardiac rhythm is crucial to the management of cardiac emergencies. An electronic rhythm generator may be connected to suitably designed manikins to enable arrhythmias to be simulated. The digitised electrocardiographic signal from the device may be monitored through chest electrodes or from the manikin chest studs that are used for defibrillation. Basic models provide the minimum requirements of sinus rhythm and the rhythms responsible for cardiac arrest (ventricular fibrillation, ventricular tachycardia, and asystole). More advanced models provide a wide range of arrhythmias, and the heart rate, rhythm, or QRST morphology may be changed instantly by the instructor, who therefore remains in control of the simulated cardiac arrest. The device may be programmed to change rhythm after the delivery of a direct current shock so that students may actually monitor the effects of defibrillation in a lifelike way. It should be remembered that energies of 50–400 J are associated with potentially lethal voltages of 2·5–7 kV, and the specially designed manikin defibrillation skin that incorporates an attenuator box must always be used.

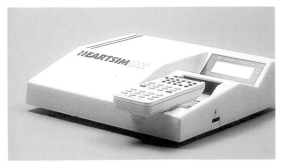

Laerdal Heart Sim 2000 enables simulation of a wide range of cardiac rhythms.

Further authenticity is provided by some manikins which produce a palpable pulse when the electrocadiographic rhythm changes to one consistent with a viable cardiac output.

Intravenous access

Several models currently available enable practice in peripheral or central venous cannulation. A plastic skin overlies the "veins," which are simulated by plastic tubes containing coloured liquid. The skin provides a realistic impression of cutaneous resistance while the veins provide further resistance to the needle; once the vein is entered the coloured fluid can be aspirated. Some models permit the placement of intravenous catheters by the Seldinger or catheter through cannula technique. Manikins are available that allow peripheral venous cannulation in several different sites. Manikins for central venous cannulation allow access to the subclavian and jugular veins; these feature the appropriate anatomical landmarks, and some incorporate a compressible bulb that enables the instructor to simulate nearby arterial pulsation.

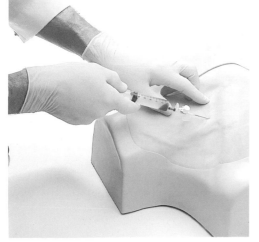

Manikin for practising a central venous cannulation.

The future

The range of "spontaneous" responses is restricted in most current manikins. There is a need for automated respiratory and circulatory activity and for controllable clinical responses such as changes in pupil size and cerebral responsiveness that enable the trainee to monitor the progress of a resuscitation attempt in a lifelike manner.

Manufacturers and Distributors

Adam Rouilly (London) Ltd, Crown Quay Lane, Sittingbourne, Kent ME10 3JG. Telephone 01795 471378 Fax 01795 479787

Ambu International (UK) Ltd, Charlton Road, Midsomer Norton, Bath BA3 4DR. Telephone 01761 416868 Fax 01761 419429

Drager Medical, The Willows, Mark Road, Hemel Hempstead, Hertfordshire HP2 7BW. Telephone 01442 213542 Fax 01442 240327

Laerdal Medical Ltd, Laerdal House, Goodmead Road, Orpington, Kent BR6 0HX. Telephone 01689 876634 Fax 01689 873800

Further reading

Emergency Care Research Institute. Training manikins, CPR. *Health Devices* 1981; **10**: 227–53.

Simons RS. Training aids and models. In: Baskett PJF, ed. *Cardiopulmonary resuscitation*. Amsterdam: Elsevier Biomedical Press, 1989; 347–83.

Committee for Evaluation of Sanitary Practices in CPR Training. Recommendations for decontaminating manikins used in cardiopulmonary resuscitation training. *Respiratory Care* 1984; **29**: 1250–2.

17 THE ETHICS OF RESUSCITATION

Peter J F Baskett

Present day knowledge, skill, pharmacy, and technology have proved effective in prolonging useful life for many patients. Countless thousands have good reason to be thankful for cardiopulmonary resuscitation, and the numbers rise daily. Yet, in the wake of this advance, there is a small but important shadow of bizarre and distressing problems. These problems must be freely and openly faced if we are to avoid criticism from others and from our own consciences.

Resuscitation attempts in the mortally ill do not enhance the dignity and serenity that we hope for our relatives and ourselves when we die. All too often resuscitation is begun in patients already destined for life as cardiac or respiratory cripples or who are suffering the terminal misery of untreatable cancer. From time to time, but fortunately rarely, resuscitation efforts may help to create the ultimate tragedy, the human vegetable, as the heart is more tolerant than the brain to the insult of hypoxia.

Merely prolonging the process of dying

The reasons for these apparent errors of judgment are several. In a high proportion of cases, especially those occurring outside hospital, the victim and his or her circumstances are unknown to the rescuer, who may well not be qualified to assess whether resuscitation is appropriate or not in the particular individual. Sadly, through lack of communication, this state of affairs also occurs from time to time in hospital practice. A junior ward nurse unless explicitly instructed not to do so feels, not unreasonably, obliged to call the resuscitation team to any patient with cardiorespiratory arrest. She or he is not qualified to certify death. The team is often unaware of the patient's condition and prognosis and, because of the urgency of the situation, begin treatment first and ask questions afterwards.

Ideally, resuscitation should be attempted only in patients who have a high chance of successful revival to a comfortable and contented existence. A study of published reports containing the results of resuscitation attempts shows that this ideal is far from being attained. Typical figures include 12% one month survival rate in 1972,[1] 14% survival to hospital discharge in 1973,[2] and, more recently, a discharge rate of 14% in 1982[3] and 21.3% in 1984.[4] De Bard, reviewing published studies in 1981, reported an overall discharge rate of 17%.[5] More recent works still put overall survival rates in the general wards of hospitals at around 15%.[6-10] In each of these series a substantial number of patients—usually about 50–60%—failed to respond to the initial resuscitation attempts. In many of these, particularly the younger patients, effort was clearly justified initially; the cause of the arrest was commonly myocardial ischaemia, when the outcome cannot be

confidently predicted in any individual patient. Some of the papers, however, drew attention to the large proportion of patients in whom resuscitation efforts were inappropriate and unjustified. Sowden et al reported an incidence of 25% of cases in which resuscitation merely prolonged the process of dying.[4]

A 32 year old woman was admitted in a quadriplegic state due to a spinal injury incurred when she had thrown herself from the Clifton Suspension Bridge. She had made 18 previous attempts at suicide over the previous five years; sometimes by taking an overdose of tablets of various kinds and sometimes by cutting her wrists. She had been injecting herself with heroin for the past seven years and had no close relationship with her family and no close friends. During her stay of two days in the intensive care unit she developed pneumonia and died. A conscious decision not to provide artificial ventilation and resuscitation had been made beforehand.

Though assessments are undoubtedly easier in retrospect, there are clearly many cases in which the decision not to resuscitate might have been made before the event. As the number of deaths in hospital always exceed the number of calls for resuscitation, a decision not to resuscitate is clearly being made in many instances. There is, however, much room for improvement.

The matter has been considered by national authorities in the United States,[11] by the European Resuscitation Council,[12 13] and by the Resuscitation Council (UK) in their *Advanced life support manual.*[14] Clearly national differences exist, dictated by legal, economic, and social variables,[15] but it is apparent that non-coercive guidelines can be set out to reduce the number of futile resuscitation attempts and to offer advice as to when resuscitation should be discontinued in the unresponding patient.

Selection of patients "Not for resuscitation"

Two settings may be envisaged:
- The unexpected cardiorespiratory arrest with no other obvious underlying disease. In this setting resuscitation should be attempted without question or delay.
- The unexpected cardiorespiratory arrest in a patient with a serious underlying disease. It is the patient in this group who should be assessed beforehand as to whether a resuscitation attempt is considered appropriate or not.

The decision not to resuscitate revolves around many factors: the patient's own wishes, which may include a "living will"; the patient's prognosis both immediate and long term; the views of relatives and friends, who may be reporting the known wishes of a patient who cannot communicate; and the patient's perceived ability to cope with disablement in the environment for which he or she is destined. The decision should not revolve around the pride of any doctor.

The examples in the boxes may serve as food for thought as to whether the value judgment was right or wrong.

Decisions on whether or not to resuscitate are generally made for each patient in the atmosphere of close clinical supervision prevalent in critical care units, and the decision is then communicated to the resident medical and nursing staff. In the general wards, however, the matter may not actually be considered for certain patients; inappropriate resuscitation then occurs by default. There has been a reluctance to label a mentally alert patient, who is nevertheless terminally ill, "not for resuscitation." There are, sadly, doctors who refuse to acknowledge that their patients have reached end stage disease, perhaps because they have spent so much time and effort in treating them. There are those who, having spent their career in hospital practice, cannot comprehend the difficulties for the severely disabled of an existence without adequate help in a poor and miserable social environment. There are those who fear medicolegal sanctions if they put their name to an instruction not to resuscitate.

Fortunately current opinion is changing, and there are now few members of the public or the profession who disagree with the concept of selection of patients deemed not suitable for resuscitation.

The decision maker should be the senior doctor in charge of the patient's management. That senior doctor, however, will usually want to take into account the opinions and wishes of the patient and the relatives and the views of the junior doctors, family practitioners, and nurses who have cared for the patient before arriving at a decision.

Once the decision not to resuscitate has been made it should be clearly communicated to the medical and nursing staff on duty and recorded in the patient's notes. Because circumstances may change, the decision must be reviewed at intervals which may range from a few hours to weeks depending on the stability of the patient's condition.

A hospital ethical resuscitation policy

"Do not resuscitate" policies have been introduced in Canada and the United States.[17] They tend to be formal affairs with a strict protocol to be followed.

Nevertheless, to minimise tragedies and to improve success rates associated with resuscitation, it is helpful to establish an agreed non-coercive hospital ethical policy based on the principle of resuscitation for all except when contraindicated. The promulgation of such guidelines serves as a reminder that the decision must be faced and made.

The guidelines for such a policy should be that:
- The decision not to resuscitate should be made by a senior doctor who should consult others as appropriate
- The decision should be communicated to medical and nursing staff, recorded in the patient's notes, and reviewed at appropriate intervals
- The decision should be shared with the patient's relatives except in a few cases when this would be deemed inappropriate
- Other appropriate treatment and care should be continued.

Below is an extract from the guidelines approved by the medical staff committee at Frenchay Hospital, Bristol, which has been in use for the past eight years.

There can be no rules, every case must be considered individually and this decision should be reviewed as appropriate—this may be on a weekly, daily, or hourly basis. The decision should be made before it is needed and in many patients this will be on admission.

A decision to "DO NOT RESUSCITATE", IS ABSOLUTELY COMPATIBLE WITH CONTINUING MAXIMUM THERAPEUTIC AND NURSING CARE.

(1) Where the patient is competent (ie mentally fit and conscious), the decision "DO NOT RESUSCITATE" should be discussed where possible with the patient. This will not always be appropriate but, particularly in those patients with a slow progressive deterioration, it is important to consider it.

(2) If the patient is not competent to make such decisions, the appropriate family members should be consulted.

(3) Factors which may influence the decision to be made should include:-
   (a) Quality of life prior to this illness (highly subjective and only truly known to the patient himself).
   (b) Expected quality of life (medical and social) assuming recovery from this particular illness.
   (c) Likelihood of resuscitation being successful.

If at any time patients or their relatives request an attempt at resuscitation contrary to medical opinion—this should be carried out.

The decision to "DO NOT RESUSCITATE" should be recorded clearly in medical and nursing notes, signed, dated, and should be reviewed at appropriate intervals.

During its period of clinical use there have been no objections to the guidelines from either the medical or nursing staff.

Termination of resuscitation attempts

If resuscitation does not result in a fairly early return of spontaneous circulation then one of two options must be considered: termination of further resuscitation efforts and support of the circulation by mechanical means such as cardiac pacing, balloon pumping, or cardiopulmonary bypass.

The decision to terminate resuscitative efforts will depend on a number of factors:

The environment and access to emergency medical services—Cardiac arrest occurring in remote sites when access to these services is impossible or delayed is not associated with a favourable outcome.

The interval between the onset of cardiac arrest and the application of basic life support—This is crucial in determining whether the outcome will include intact neurological function. Generally speaking if the interval between cardiac arrest and the start of cardiopulmonary resuscitation is greater than 5 minutes the prognosis is poor except in special cases such as hypothermia or previous intake of a sedative drug; children also tend to be more tolerant of delay.

The interval between basic life support and the application of advanced life support measures—Survival is rare if defibrillation or drug treatment, or both, is not available within 30 minutes of cardiac arrest. Each case must be judged on individual merit, taking into account evidence of cardiac death, cerebral damage, and the ultimate prognosis.

Evidence of cardiac death—Persistent ventricular fibrillation should continue to be actively treated until established asystole or electromechanical dissociation (pulseless electrical activity) supervenes. Patients with asystole who are unresponsive to adrenaline and fluid replacement are unlikely to survive except in special circumstances (for example, hypothermia or drug overdose) and resuscitation should be abandoned after 15 minutes.

Evidence of cerebral damage—Fixed and dilated pupils, unrelated to previous drug treatment, are usually (but not invariably) an indication of serious cerebral damage, and consideration should be given to abandoning resuscitation in the absence of mitigating factors. If the measurement system is in place, intracranial pressure values greater than 30 mmHg are a poor prognostic sign.

Potential prognosis and underlying disease process—Resuscitation should be abandoned early when patients have a poor ultimate prognosis or end stage disease. Prolonged attempts in such patients are rarely successful and are associated with a high risk of cerebral damage.

Age has less effect on outcome than the underlying disease process[7] or the presenting cardiac rhythm.[4] Nevertheless, patients in their 70s and 80s do not have good survival rates compared with younger subjects, generally because of underlying disease,[16] and earlier curtailment of resuscitation is indicated. By contrast, young children seem to be tolerant of hypoxia, and resuscitation should be continued for longer than for adults.

Temperature—Hypothermia confers protection against the effects of hypoxia and therefore resuscitation efforts should be continued for much longer than in normothermic patients. Cases have been reported of survival with good neurological function after more than one hour's submersion in cold water. Resuscitation should be continued in hypothermic patients during active rewarming by using cardiopulmonary bypass if available and appropriate.

Drug intake before cardiac arrest—Sedative, hypnotic, or narcotic drugs taken before cardiac arrest also provide a degree of cerebral protection against the effects of hypoxia and resuscitative efforts should be prolonged accordingly.

Remediable precipitating factors—Resuscitation should continue while potentially remediable conditions are treated. Such conditions include tension pneumothorax and cardiac tamponade. Outcome after cardiac arrest due to haemorrhagic hypovolaemia is notoriously poor. Factors to be taken into account include the immediate availability of skilled surgery and rapid transfusion facilities. Even under optimal conditions survival rates are poor, and early termination of resuscitation is generally indicated if bleeding cannot be immediately controlled.

Other resuscitation procedures

Use of cardiac pacing

Cardiac pacing (internal or transthoracic) has limited application after cardiac arrest. Pacing should be reserved for those patients with recognisable electrical activity on the electrocardiogram or with symptomatic bradycardia.

Balloon pump and cardiopulmonary bypass

The use of these techniques will clearly depend on the immediate availability of the necessary equipment and skilled staff. Such intervention should be reserved for patients with a potentially good prognosis—for instance, cases of hypothermia, drug overdose, and those with conditions amenable to immediate cardiac, thoracic, or abdominal surgery.

Legal aspects

Doctors, nurses, and paramedical staff functioning in their official capacity have an obligation to perform cardiopulmonary resuscitation when medically indicated and in the absence of a "do not resuscitate" decision.

Many countries apply "Good Samaritan" laws in relation to cardiopulmonary resuscitation to protect lay rescuers acting in good faith, provided they are not guilty of gross negligence. In other countries the law may not be specifically written down, but the Good Samaritan principle is applied by the judiciary. Such arrangements are essential for the creation and continuance of a community and hospital cardiopulmonary resuscitation policy. At the time of writing, I do not know of any case in which a lay person has been successfully sued after making a reasonable attempt at cardiopulmonary resuscitation. Similar protection applies to teachers and trainers of citizen cardiopulmonary resuscitation programmes.

Health care professionals, outside their place of work and acting as bystander citizens, are expected to perform basic cardiopulmonary resuscitation only within the limitations of the environment and facilities available to them on the occasion.

When acting in their employed capacities, health care professionals are expected to be able to perform basic life support, and all doctors are expected additionally to provide the major elements of advanced life support, including airway management, ventilation with oxygen, defibrillation, intravenous cannulation, and appropriate drug treatment. Hospitals are expected to provide resuscitation equipment and facilities. With increasing expectation of higher standards it is likely that these requirements will be extended in the future to family medical and dental practices, leisure, sports, and travel centres, trains, planes, ships, and places of work.

The status of "do not resuscitate" policies is rarely defined precisely in the legislature of most European countries. The majority of the judiciary, however, accept in practice a decision not to resuscitate, carefully arrived at and based on the guidelines outlined above.

A 62 year old woman had a cardiac arrest in a thoracic ward two days after undergoing pneumonectomy for resectable lung cancer. Her remaining lung was clearly fibrotic and malfunctioning, and her cardiac arrest was probably hypoxic and hypercarbic in origin. Because no instructions had been given to the contrary, she was resuscitated by the hospital resuscitation team and spontaneous cardiac rhythm restarted after 20 minutes. She required continuous artificial ventilation and was unconscious for a week. Over the next six weeks she gradually regained consciousness but could not be weaned from the ventilator. She was tetraplegic—presumably as a result of spinal cord damage from hypoxia—but regained some weak finger movement over two months. At three months her improvement had tailed off, and she was virtually paralysed in all four limbs and dependent on the ventilator. She died five months after the cardiac arrest. She was supported throughout the illness by her devoted and intelligent husband, who left his work to be with her and continued to hope for a spontaneous cure until very near the end.

Infection hazards during resuscitation

Mouth to mouth ventilation

Cross infection between victim and rescuer may potentially occur during mouth to mouth or mouth to nose ventilation. The incidence is remarkably low, but isolated cases of cutaneous tuberculosis, herpes labialis, staphylococcal and streptococcal infections, and meningococcal meningitis have been reported.

Of great concern to would be rescuers at the present time is the possibility of acquiring HIV infection during mouth to mouth contact. Fortunately is seems that HIV is not contained in saliva in amounts sufficient to cause infection[17] but there always remains the possibility of transmission from open oral wounds in either the victim or rescuer. At the time of writing there is, however, no record of this ever having occurred and so the possibility must be considered almost non-existent. The chance of infection with the hepatitis B virus is, however, greater.

On the evidence currently available it is reasonable to encourage would be rescuers in the community to continue to perform unprotected mouth to mouth ventilation in patients with cardiorespiratory arrest with the assurance that the risk of infection is negligible. Any one lay person is unlikely to perform cardiopulmonary resuscitation more than six times in a lifetime, and there is a 75% chance that resuscitation will be given to a relative, close friend, or a workmate. Nevertheless, small simple protective plastic film devices (for example, Ambu Life Key and Laerdal Resusci Face Shield) are available to prevent direct contact; the use of these by lay bystanders is to be encouraged if they are immediately available. Resuscitation should never be delayed, however, while the equipment is sought.

Health care professionals have a much higher chance of being called on to perform resuscitation, and it is therefore reasonable that protective devices should be readily available in each patient area to offer protection against infection and to reduce aesthetic antagonism. The Laerdal Pocket Mask is one of the most satisfactory devices for this purpose. Similar devices are made by other manufacturers.

Blood to blood contact

Advanced life support often entails an invasive procedure. It is good practice for all professional rescuers to wear protective gloves throughout. Special care should be taken to minimise needle stick injuries and cuts from ampoules. Disposal boxes for "sharps" should be immediately available. Goggles should also be worn, particularly when patients are thought to represent special risks.

Training manikins

Training manikins have not been shown in practice to be a source of viral infection for resuscitation students. Nevertheless, the potential for bacterial infections does exist, and it is good practice to disinfect the equipment after each use according to the manufacturers' instructions.

Other ethical problems arising in relation to resuscitation

There are several other unsolved ethical problems arising in relation to resuscitation which need to be dealt with.

The diagnosis of death

Traditionally, death is pronounced by medical practitioners. The question, however, arises as to the wisdom and practicality in some cases of death being determined by non-medical health care professionals, such as nurses or ambulance staff.

Such a policy might obviate the need for futile or excessively prolonged resuscitation attempts. Certainly there would be no argument in straightforward cases such as decapitation, incineration, prolonged submersion, and massive mutilation. The question also arises, however, in cases of extreme senility and terminal illness when no previous medical instructions have been given and in patients who are unresponsive to prolonged resuscitation attempts outside hospital. This subject is currently under debate by authorities in the United Kingdom and other countries.

Involvement of relatives and close friends

Bystanders are being actively encouraged to undertake immediate basic life support in the event of cardiorespiratory arrest. In many cases the bystander will be a close relative. Traditionally relatives are escorted away from the victim when the health care professionals arrive. It is clear, however, that some relatives do not wish to be isolated from their loved one at this time and are deeply hurt if this is insisted on. Aspects of this debate have been published with contributions from a relative and members of the medical profession[18]; opinion confirms the need to identify and respect relatives' wishes to remain with the patient. Care and consideration for the relative in these stressful situations becomes of increasing concern as the invasiveness of the resuscitation escalates from basic life support, to defibrillation and venous access, and perhaps to chest drainage, cricothyrotomy, and even open chest cardiac massage.

The use of the recently dead for training in practical skills

Opportunities for hands on training in the practical skills required for resuscitation are limited. It is clear that tracheal intubation cannot be taught to everyone attending a cardiac arrest, and while the laryngeal mask may offer an alternative option for airway management in the short term, the introduction of that device on a widespread scale into anaesthetic practice has, in itself, reduced the opportunities for training in the anaesthetic room. Manikin training offers an alternative, but most would agree that training on patients is required to amplify manikin experience. Training in tracheal intubation on the recently dead has engendered a sharp debate and, while supported by some doctors, has met with strong opposition from members of the nursing profession. Informed consent is difficult to obtain at the sensitive and emotional time of bereavement and approaches may be construed as coercion. On the other hand proceeding without consent may constitute assault.

The dilemma does not stop with tracheal intubation, and other techniques such as fibreoptic intubation, central venous access, surgical cut down venous access, chest drain insertion, and surgical cricothyrotomy should be considered.

Modern medicine brings problems and ethical dilemmas. Public expectations have changed and will continue to change. More and more, doctors' actions are questioned in the media and in the courts of law. We need to formulate answers and be more open with the public in explaining how our actions are related entirely to their wellbeing. Only in this way will we keep in tune with society and practise the science of resuscitation with art and compassion.

1 Wildsmith JAW, Denyson WG, Myers KW. Results of resuscitation following cardiac arrest. *Br J Anaesth* 1972; 44: 716–9.
2 Eltringham RJ, Baskett PJF. Experience with a hospital resuscitation service including an analysis of 258 calls to patients with cardiorespiratory arrest. *Resuscitation* 1973; 2: 57–68.
3 Hershey CO, Fisher L. Why outcome of cardiopulmonary resuscitation in general wards is so poor. *Lancet* 1982; ii: 32.
4 Sowden GR, Baskett PJF, Robins DW. Factors associated with survival and eventual cerebral status following cardiac arrest. *Anaesthesia* 1984; 39: 1.
5 De Bard ML. Cardiopulmonary resuscitation: analysis of six years experience and review of the literature. *Ann Emerg Med* 1981; 10: 408–16.
6 Council on Ethical and Judicial Affairs, American Heart Association. Guidelines for the appropriate use of do-not-resuscitate orders. *JAMA* 1991; 265: 1968–71.
7 Bedell SE, Delbanco TL, Cook EF, Epstein FH. Survival after cardiopulmonary resuscitation in hospital. *N Engl J Med* 1983; 309: 569–76.

8 Evans AL, Brody BA. The do not resuscitate order in teaching hospitals. *JAMA* 1985; **253**: 2236–9.

9 Moss AH. Informing the patient about cardiopulmonary resuscitation: when the risks outweigh the benefits. *J Gen Intern Med* 1989; **4**: 349–55.

10 Tunstall Pedoe H, Bailey L, Chamberlain DA, Marsden AK, Ward ME. Zideman DA. Survey of 3765 cardiopulmonary resuscitations in British Hospitals. The BRESUS study: methods and overall results. *BMJ* 1992; **304**: 1347–51.

11. American Heart Association; Emergency Cardiac Care Committee. Guidelines for cardiopulmonary resuscitation and emergency cardiac care. Ethical considerations in resuscitation. *JAMA* 1992; **268**: 2282–8.

12 Baskett PJF. Ethics in cardiopulmonary resuscitation (Invited Editorial). *Resuscitation* 1993; **25**: 1, 8.

13 Holmberg S, Ekstrom L. Ethics and practicalities of resuscitation. *Resuscitation* 1992; **24**: 239–44.

14 Resuscitation Council UK. *Advanced life support manual.* Handley AJ, ed. London: Resuscitation Council UK, 1992.

15 Bossaert L. Ethical issues in resuscitation. In: J L Vincent, ed. *Yearbook of intensive care and emergency medicine.* Berlin, Springer Verlag, 1994: 408–15.

16 Ritter G, Wolfe RA, Goldstein S, Landis JR, Vash CM, Acheson A, Leighton R, Medendrop SV. The effect by bystander CPR on survival of out of hospital cardiac arrest victims. *Am Heart J* 1985; **110**: 932–37.

17 Center for Disease Control. Update: universal precautions for prevention of transmission of human immunodeficiency virus, hepatitis B virus and other blood borne pathogens in health care settings. *MMWR* 1988; **37**: 377–88.

18 Adams S, Whitlock M, Higgs R, Bloomfield P and Baskett PJF. Should relatives be allowed to watch resuscitation. *BMJ* 1994; **308**: 1687–9.

18 DRUGS AND THEIR DELIVERY

Michael C Colquhoun

The role of drugs in resuscitation from cardiopulmonary arrest has undergone considerable revision in recent years. Advances in the understanding of their pharmacology have enabled a more rational approach to be made to their use. An important principal behind current recommendations is that drugs should be used only when there is real evidence of their worth.

In this chapter the main classes of drugs used are considered as well as the routes by which they may be administered.

Routes of drug delivery

During resuscitation attempts most drugs are given by the intravenous or endobronchial routes, but the intraosseous route is occasionally used, particularly in children. Intracardiac injection, although previously popular, should now be considered only as a last resort, if at all.

Intravenous routes

Peripheral venous cannulation is safe, easily learnt, and does not require interruption of cardiopulmonary resuscitation. It may, however, be difficult in hypovolaemic or obese patients. A large vein, usually in the antecubital fossa, is the site of choice. Once a cannula is in place it should be connected to an intravenous infusion which can be run in rapidly to aid drug administration. Raising the limb and massaging the veins will speed delivery to the central circulation.

Central venous cannulation enables drugs to reach their sites of action more rapidly, but the technique requires greater skill. It is particularly useful when poor peripheral perfusion makes cannulation of veins technically difficult. The internal jugular and subclavian are the veins most often used. It should be remembered, however, that subclavian access requires interruption of chest compression while internal jugular cannulation may interfere with ventilation. Complications of the technique include haemorrhage, arterial puncture, pneumothorax, and extravascular drug administration. Thrombolytic drugs should not subsequently be given through central vein cannulas inserted during resuscitation because of the risk of local haemorrhage.

Endobronchial route

Tracheal intubation is often performed at an early stage during resuscitation particularly outside hospital, and the endobronchial route is therefore often the first one available for the administration of drugs. Adrenaline, atropine, and lignocaine can be given by this route; the recommended doses are double those given intravenously. The drugs should be diluted to a total volume of 10 ml with isotonic saline and injected through a catheter passed beyond the tip of the tracheal tube; their rate of absorption will depend on the efficiency of cardiopulmonary resuscitation and will be reduced in the presence of pulmonary oedema. Conflicting evidence about the efficiency of this method of drug administration has been reported from clinical and experimental studies, and it cannot be considered the route of first choice.

Intraosseous route

The bone marrow in the tibia consists of a venous plexus which drains directly into the central circulation. Drugs may be given through a special intraosseous cannula inserted into the tibia proximal to the medial maleolus. This technique is particularly valuable in children, although limited reports of its use in adults have also been favourable. Adrenaline, atropine, and lignocaine can be given by the intraosseous route preferably as an infusion; the doses are the same as for the intravenous route.

Intracardiac injection

Injection is normally into the right ventricle, either via the subxiphoid approach or through the fifth left intercostal space. It requires considerable skill, however, to perform these injections accurately, and postmortem studies have shown that often the drug is not given into the heart at all. Damage to the myocardium and coronary arteries is common, and other complications include haemothorax, pneumothorax, and haemopericardium. Intracardiac injections should be considered only as a last resort when no other route is available.

Drugs used in resuscitation attempts
Catecholamine and vasopressor drugs

Vasopressor drugs are used during cardiopulmonary resuscitation to produce peripheral vasoconstriction and thereby raise systemic vascular resistance. Coronary blood flow during closed chest cardiopulmonary resuscitation is determined by the pressure gradient across the myocardium (that is, the difference between aortic and right atrial pressure). By causing vasoconstriction in the peripheral circulation catecholamines raise the aortic pressure thereby increasing coronary perfusion. Differential shunting of blood to the coronary and cerebral circulation also occurs.

Adrenaline (epinephrine) is the drug currently recommended in the management of all three forms of cardiac arrest (see chapters 2 and 3). It stimulates $\alpha 1$, $\alpha 2$, $\beta 1$, and $\beta 2$ receptors, but it is the effect on the α receptors that is beneficial. β stimulation may be detrimental as $\beta 1$ stimulation increases heart rate and force of contraction (thereby raising myocardial oxygen requirements) and $\beta 2$ stimulation increases glycogenolysis (with increased oxygen requirements) and produces hypokalaemia (with increased chance of arrhythmia). To avoid the potentially detrimental β effects, selective $\alpha 1$ agonists have been investigated but have been found to be ineffective in most settings.

Within the vascular smooth muscle of the peripheral resistance vessels both $\alpha 1$ and $\alpha 2$ receptors produce vasoconstriction. During hypoxic states it is thought that the $\alpha 1$ receptors become less potent and that the $\alpha 2$ adrenergic receptors contribute more towards vasomotor tone. This may explain the ineffectiveness of pure $\alpha 1$ agonists; adrenaline and noradrenaline, which possess both $\alpha 1$ and $\alpha 2$ agonist action, have been shown to enhance coronary perfusion pressure considerably during cardiac arrest. The α 2 agonist activity seems to become increasingly important as the duration of circulatory arrest progresses, and the β agonist activity (which both drugs possess) seems to work at least partly beneficially by counteracting α 2 agonist mediated coronary vasoconstriction.

Several clinical trials have compared different vasopressor agents in the treatment of cardiac arrest, but none has been shown to be more effective than adrenaline, which therefore remains the drug of choice. Although work on animals has suggested potential haemodynamic advantages for larger doses of adrenaline than those currently used, clinical trials have not shown a clear benefit. For example, a dose of adrenaline of 5 mg in patients with asystole and electromechanical dissociation was associated with a higher initial resuscitation rate when compared with a dose of 1 mg, but the hospital discharge rate was not improved. Detrimental effects of high catecholamine concentrations include sustained myocardial contraction and necrosis, increased myocardial oxygen demands in ventricular fibrillation, coronary vasoconstriction, hypertension after successful resuscitation, and an increase in systemic oxygen consumption. The standard dose of adrenaline therefore remains 1 mg.

Atropine

Atropine antagonises the parasympathetic neurotransmitter acetylcholine at muscarinic receptors. The most important effects are on the vagus nerve; by lowering vagal tone on the heart, sinus node automaticity is increased and atrioventricular conduction is augmented. Increased parasympathetic tone, for example after myocardial infarction, may lead to bradyarrythymias including asystole, and atropine is effective treatment in this setting. When increased parasympathetic tone in the peripheral vascular system contributes to hypotension atropine may also be useful.

Atropine has been widely used in the treatment of asystole, but the drug has never been proved conclusively to be of value in this situation. Asystole, however, carries a grave prognosis and there are anecdotal accounts of success after its use. Moreover, it has no important side effects and therefore should be given, once only, in a dose of 3 mg, which is adequate to block vagal tone completely.

Antiarrhythmic drugs

Antiarrhythmic drugs are used both for the prevention and treatment of cardiac arrest. Lignocaine is the one that has been studied most extensively. It has been used to treat ventricular tachycardia and fibrillation and to prevent recurrences of these arrhythmias after successful resuscitation. It has also been used as an adjunct to defibrillation in cases resistant to direct current shock. Several trials have shown that lignocaine is effective in preventing ventricular fibrillation after acute myocardial infarction, but no reduction in mortality has been shown, probably because the trials were conducted in a setting where defibrillation was readily available to reverse ventricular fibrillation in all patients.

Data about the effectiveness of lignocaine in preventing arrhythmias have been extrapolated to suggest that it may also be effective in the treatment of ventricular fibrillation, particularly when used as an adjunct to defibrillation. Studies on animals, however, have consistently shown that the energy required for defibrillation is actually increased when lignocaine is used, and in one clinical trial in human subjects there was a threefold greater occurrence of asystole after defibrillation when lignocaine had been given.

Bretylium is a complex drug possessing antiarrhythmic activity that has also been investigated in an attempt to find a pharmacological adjunct to defibrillation. Unfortunately its antiarrhythmic action takes a considerable time to become established and basic life support must be continued for at least 20 minutes after its administration. To date, randomised prospective trials comparing lignocaine with bretylium have not produced clear cut results.

Amiodarone is certainly effective in preventing ventricular arrhythmias; it has proved successful in cases resistant to other drugs and in the treatment of patients at high risk of sudden death from lethal arrhythmias. Animal studies suggest that amiodarone can reduce the defibrillation threshold, and this has been confirmed in one human study, but there has been no experimental work directly applicable to the setting that exists in most resuscitation attempts. Randomised prospective studies of lignocaine, bretylium, and amiodarone (and placebo) are urgently required.

Calcium

Calcium has a vital role in cardiac excitation-contraction coupling mechanisms and has been recommended for the treatment of electromechanical dissociation, despite a lack of supporting scientific evidence. There is in fact now considerable evidence to suggest that its use during cardiac arrest is ineffective and possibly harmful.

Neither serum nor tissue calcium concentrations fall after cardiac arrest; bolus injections of a calcium salt will raise intracellular calcium concentrations and may produce myocardial necrosis or uncontrolled contracture. Smooth muscle in peripheral arteries may also contract in the presence of high calcium concentrations further reducing blood flow; the brain is particularly susceptible and calcium antagonists have been reported to improve cerebral recovery.

On the basis of the evidence from animal work and clinical studies the use of calcium in electromechanical dissociation or asystole is not recommended except in known cases of hypocalaemia, hyperkalaemia, or where calcium antagonists have been given. In practice it may be uncertain whether these conditions exist in an individual patient, and it seems reasonable to continue to use calcium as a last resort in a desperate situation.

Alkalising agents

During cardiac arrest gaseous exchange in the lungs ceases while cellular metabolism continues in an anaerobic environment; this produces a combination of respiratory and metabolic acidosis. The most effective treatment for this condition (until the spontaneous circulation can be restored) is chest compression to maintain the circulation, and ventilation to provide oxygen and remove carbon dioxide.

Sodium bicarbonate

In the past, infusion of sodium bicarbonate has been advocated early in the course of management of cardiac arrest in an attempt to reverse acidosis. The action of sodium bicarbonate as a buffer agent depends on the ability of the lungs to remove the carbon dioxide generated.

Every 1 mmol of carbon dioxide produced in the buffering action of bicarbonate generates 22·4 ml of gaseous carbon dioxide; this greatly increases the partial pressure of carbon dioxide in the blood. Severe respiratory

Drugs and their delivery

acidosis results as circulatory failure limits the ability of the lungs to excrete the carbon dioxide. One further effect of hypercarbia is a paradoxical intracellular acidosis because carbon dioxide diffuses rapidly into cells; the effects may be particularly clear in the brain, which lacks the phosphate and protein buffers found in other tissues. Accumulation of carbon dioxide in the myocardium causes further depression of myocardial contractility. Sodium bicarbonate solution is hyperosmolar in the concentrations usually used, and the sodium load may exacerbate cerebral oedema. In the experimental setting hyperosmolality has been correlated with reduced aortic pressure and reduced coronary perfusion in consequence.

Only judicious use of sodium bicarbonate can be recommended, and correction of acidosis should be based on determinations of pH and base excess. Arterial blood is not suitable for this measurement; central venous blood samples better reflect tissue acidosis.

There is no generally agreed level of acidosis at which sodium bibarbonate should be considered, but a pH of less than 7·0–7·1 with a base excess of less than -10 has been recommended. Units of no more than 40–50 milli equivalents (or 0·5–0·7 milliequivalents per kg body weight) is the maximum recommended dose. Sodium bicarbonate may also be indicated when hyperkalaemia or metabolic acidosis are known to be present at the time of cardiac arrest.

The return of spontaneous circulation and adequate ventilation is the best way to ensure correction of the acid base disturbances that accompany cardiopulmonary arrest.

Alternatives to sodium bicarbonate

Several agents have been suggested as alternatives to the traditional sodium bicarbonate; tris hydroxymethyl aminomethane (THAN), calcicarb (equimolar combination of sodium bicarbonate and sodium carbonate), and tribonate (a combination of THAN, sodium acetate, sodium bicarbonate, and sodium phosphate) have been recommended. They have the advantage of producing little or no carbon dioxide, but animal studies have not shown consistent benefits over sodium bicarbonate and further investigation is required before the place of these agents is established.

Pharmacological approaches to cerebral protection after cardiac arrest

The cerebral ischaemia that follows cardiac arrest results in the rapid exhaustion of cerebral oxygen, glucose, and high energy phosphates. Cell membranes start to leak almost immediately and cerebral oedema results. Calcium channels in the cell membrane open and there is an influx of calcium into the cell which is thought to trigger a cascade of events resulting in neuronal damage. If resuscitation is successful reperfusion of the cerebral circulation can itself further damage nerve cells. Several mechanisms for this have been proposed including vasospasm, red cell sludging, hypermetabolic states, and acidosis.

Early attempts at cerebral protection aimed at reproducing the depression in brain metabolism seen in hypothermia and barbiturate anaesthesia was investigated for this purpose. Although at first showing promise, several large studies have failed to confirm any benefit.

Treatment of cerebral oedema

Cerebral oedema is often present in the period after resuscitation. This is not usually regarded as a major problem, and intracranial pressure is not usually elevated. Pharmacological measures to reduce cerebral oedema have not been shown to be beneficial and the routine use of diuretics for this purpose cannot be recommended. Likewise, corticosteroids have not been shown to help, and in experimental studies their administration has resulted in considerably increased damage from cerebral ischaemia. The risks of infection, gastric haemorrhage, and elevated blood glucose concentration with steroids provide additional reasons to restrict their use.

Calcium channel blockers

Because of the role of calcium in causing neuronal injury, calcium channel blocking agents have been investigated for their possible protective effect both in animal experiments and in several clinical trials. Unfortunately none of the agents tried, including lidoflazine, nimodipine, flunarizine, and nicardepine, have been found to be beneficial. Several different calcium entry channels exist and only the voltage dependant L type are blocked by the drugs studied, therefore excess calcium entry may not have been prevented under the trial conditions.

Excitatory amino acid receptor antagonists

Recently the excitatory amino acid neurotransmitters (especially glutamate and aspartate) have been implicated in causing neuronal necrosis after ischaemia. The N-methyl-D-aspartate (NMDA) receptor, which has a role in controlling calcium influx into the cell, has been studied but unfortunately no striking benefit from specific NMDA receptor antagonists has been seen.

Free radicals

Oxygen derived free radicals have been implicated in the production of ischaemic neuronal damage. During both ischaemia and reperfusion the natural free radical scavengers are depleted. In certain experimental settings exogenous free radical scavengers (desferrioxamine, superoxide dismutase, and catalase) have been shown to influence an ischaemic insult to the brain, suggesting a potential use for these agents, although no clear role has currently been defined.

Further reading

von Planter M, Chamberlain D. Drug treatment of arrhythmias during cardiopulmonary resuscitation. *Resuscitation* 1992; **194**: 227–32.
Koster R, Carli P. Acid base management. *Resuscitation* 1992; 24: 143–6.
Hapnes SA, Robertson C. CPR–drug delivery routes and systems. *Resuscitation* 1992; 24: 137–42.
Lindner KH, Kosta R. Vasopressor drugs during cardiopulmonary resuscitation. *Resuscitation* 1992; 24: 147–53.
Chamberlain DA. Lignocaine and bretylium as adjuncts to electrical defibrillation. *Resuscitation* 1991; 22: 153–7.
Waller DG. Treatment and prevention of ventricular fibrillation: are there better agents? *Resuscitation* 1991; 22: 159–66.
Evans TR, Morgenson L. Pharmacological treatment of asystole and electromechanical dissociation. *Resuscitation* 1991; 22: 167–72.
Kripps T, Camm AJ. The management of electromechanical dissociation. *Resuscitation* 1991; 22: 173–83.
Waller DG, Robertson CE. Role of sympathomimetic amines during cardiopulmonary resuscitation. *Resuscitation* 1991; 22: 181–90.
Aitkenhead AR. Drug administration during CPR. *Resuscitation* 1991; 22: 191–5.
Aitkenhead AR. Cerebral protection after cardiac arrest. *Resuscitation* 1991; 22: 197–202.
Gustafson I, Edgren E, Multing J. Brain orientated intensive care after resuscitation from cardiac arrest. *Resuscitation* 1992; 24: 245–61.
Stueven HA, Thompson B, Aprahamian C, et al. The effectiveness of calcium chloride in refractory electromechanical dissociation. *Ann Emerg Med* 1985; **14**: 626–9.
Stueven HA, Thompson B, Aprahamian C, et al. Lack of effectiveness of calcium chloride in refractory asystole. *Ann Emerg Med* 1985; **14**: 630–3.
Brain Resuscitation Clinical Trial 1 Study Group. Randomized clinical study of thiopental loading in comatose survivors of cardiac arrest. *N Engl J Med* 1986; **314**: 397–403.

19 POSTRESUSCITATION CARE

Anthony D Redmond

Full recovery from cardiac arrest is rarely immediate. The restoration of electrocardiographic complexes marks the start and not the end of a successful resuscitation attempt. The true end point is a fully conscious, neurologically intact patient with a spontaneous stable cardiac rhythm and an adequate urine output.

The chances of achieving this are greatly enhanced if the conditions in the box are met.

Once spontaneous cardiac output has been restored ensure that a senior doctor is summoned and makes a decision about transferring the patient to an intensive care area. Elective ventilation is often necessary, and such decisions require experience and authority. If the time from the onset of cardiac arrest to return of full consciousness is about two to three minutes elective ventilation may prove unnecessary. Unfortunately this is rare and likely to occur only when the patient was already under intensive care and resuscitation was initiated with minimal delay. On a general hospital ward, although cardiac arrest is often witnessed, it may be many minutes before definitive treatment can be started. These patients will invariably need transfer to an intensive care unit for further assessment, monitoring, and treatment.

> **Successful resuscitation**
>
> Arrest was witnessed
>
> Underlying arrhythmia was ventricular fibrillation
>
> Successful cardioversion achieved in 2–3 minutes and not longer than 8 minutes
>
> When defibrillation was delayed for longer than 2–3 minutes cardiopulmonary resuscitation was started and maintained

Cerebral protection

Accident and emergency departments receive patients who have had unwitnessed arrests. In these patients special attention must be given to cerebral resuscitation. All doctors should be aware of the consequences when resuscitation is incomplete and brain damage occurs. Nevertheless, more brains are damaged by inadequate than by inappropriate resuscitation. Experienced senior doctors must be involved early in the management of cardiac arrest, ideally from the start.

When the heart stops the brain may be damaged both by the initial ischaemia and by failure of adequate reperfusion; the latter is ultimately the more damaging. The brain may survive a period of hypoxia if cerebral blood flow is maintained, but when it ceases the electroencephalogram becomes flat within 10 seconds and cerebral glucose is used up within one minute. Neuronal activity may continue for up to an hour, but unfortunately progressive deterioration of the brain cannot be reversed or halted after about three minutes of arrested circulation. A carotid pulse may be restored, but the myriad of tiny cerebral vessels cannot be reperfused. Several factors cause cerebral damage.

Vasospasm—Movement of calcium ions is implicated in vasospasm, and calcium antagonists have improved survival in animals. The routine administration of calcium must therefore be questioned.

Cerebral oedema—Hypoxia leads to cerebral oedema, which is augmented by the high blood concentration of carbon dioxide associated with apnoea. Administration of sodium bicarbonate may release yet more carbon dioxide and compound the problem. Hyperventilation and elective lowering of the partial pressure of carbon dioxide may reduce cerebral oedema and obviate the need for bicarbonate.

Microthrombus formation and sludging—When cerebral blood flow ceases the smaller vessels silt up. Once formed these blockages cannot be removed.

> **Failure of reperfusion:**
>
> Vasopasm
> Cerebral oedema
> Microthrombi and "sludging"
>
> - Restore spontaneous cardiac output
> - Control pH, blood gases, and electrolytes
> - Electively ventilate

Postresuscitation care

Cerebral damage after cardiac arrest can be minimised by the following manoeuvres:

Rapid return of spontaneous cardiac output—Cardiopulmonary resuscitation may achieve no more than 5% of normal cerebral blood flow with minimal oxygenation. It does, however, prevent total cessation of cerebral circulation.

Meticulous control of pH, blood gases, and electrolytes in the period immediately after the arrest. In most cases this can be achieved only by elective ventilation of a sedated, paralysed patient in an intensive care unit.

The use of techniques such as barbituate coma, induced hypothermia, or even steroid treatment to protect the brain against the effects of ischaemia are, at best, of unproved efficiency.

Airway and ventilation

> **Immediately after restoration of cardiac rhythm complete this checklist**
>
> (1) With a laryngoscope ensure that the *endotracheal tube* is correctly placed in the trachea and not in the oesophagus
>
> (2) Ensure that the patient is being adequately *ventilated* with *100% oxygen*. Listen with a stethoscope and confirm adequate and equal air entry. If you suspect *pneumothorax* insert a chest drain
>
> (3) Estimate *arterial pH and gases*, preferably from an arterial sample, but use a central venous sample if necessary
>
> (4) Estimate *serum potassium*
>
> (5) Obtain a *chest radiograph*. An anteroposterior supine view is adequate
>
> (6) Insert a *urinary catheter* and measure the urinary output
>
> (7) Insert a *nasogastric tube* and aspirate the contents of the stomach
>
> (8) Obtain a *12 lead electrocardiogram*

Although spontaneous respiratory effort may return quite soon after restoration of a heart beat, it is rarely adequate and the gag reflex is usually impaired. A cuffed tracheal tube will protect the airway and facilitate positive pressure ventilation. 100% Oxygen should be used to ensure adequate oxygenation. If the patient resists the tracheal tube a decision must be made whether to use sedation. This will allow control of ventilation and correction of blood gas abnormalities.

A self inflating bag and valve, used with either a face mask or tracheal tube, is inadequate for more than a few minutes of resuscitation. The use of an oxygen reservoir will ensure high inspired oxygen concentrations, but even so concentrations of carbon dioxide will build up and lead to an increase in intracranial pressure and a deterioration in the acid-base status. A mechanical ventilator should be used.

Chest compression may be complicated by a flail chest. This can be the result of rib fracture or, more commonly, of costochrondral or sternal dislocation. Elective ventilation is mandatory in these circumstances. Do not wean a patient off a ventilator unless you know that the rib cage is intact.

Acid-base balance

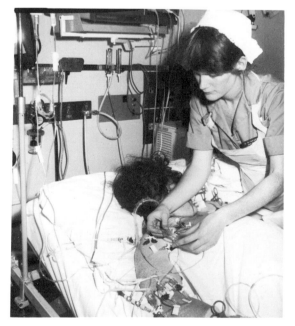

Even optimal chest compression produces poor cerebral blood flow and even less peripheral circulation. There is little effective venous return, so lactic acid builds up and is not returned to the circulation until the heart is restarted. It is in the phase immediately after recovery from cardiac arrest that serious acid-base problems may occur, and continuous monitoring of the blood gases every 15 minutes, possibly for several hours, is essential.

Blood gas and acid-base abnormalities should initially be controlled by ventilation and the restoration of renal function. If these prove inadequate then small doses of bicarbonate may be given if blood gases are constantly monitored. Sodium bicarbonate provides a large hyperosmolar sodium load to an extremely compromised circulation and can produce a precipitous fall in the serum potassium concentration. It neutralises acid by the release of carbon dioxide, and a rise in the arterial partial pressure of carbon dioxide will lead to increased cerebral oedema. Carbon dioxide will move into the cerebrospinal fluid, making central monitoring of the pH by the brain extremely precarious once cardiac output has been restored. Sodium bicarbonate should therefore never be given at the start of the procedure, must only be given to ventilated patients, and must be a response to known acid-base abnormality.

Blood electrolytes

Hypokalaemia may have precipitated cardiac arrest, particularly in elderly patients taking digoxin and diuretics. Administration of bicarbonate may then further lower the serum potassium value. If the serum potassium concentration is high, usually as the result of renal failure, then it can be lowered with glucose and insulin.

Chest x ray examination

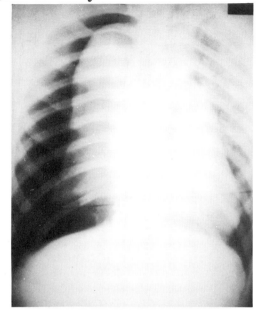

After a successful attempt at resuscitation a chest x ray photograph must be taken. From this one can check the position of the central venous line and ensure that the tracheal tube has not entered a main bronchus. A pneumothorax may have occurred and is an important reversible cause of electromechanical dissociation. Cardiac tamponade may be diagnosed by an enlarged cardiac shadow and a raised central venous pressure; if in doubt obtain an echocardiogram.

Haemodynamic assessment

The haemodynamics of the period after cardiac arrest are complex, and measurements must be made if treatment is to be safe and effective. Palpation of the pulse and listening for Korotkoff sounds in the arm does not constitute assessment of the haemodynamics. A high systemic vascular resistance in a low flow state will prevent Korotkoff sounds being heard, despite a relatively high mean arterial pressure. Indwelling pulmonary and systemic arterial catheters must be inserted to measure the true haemodynamic state before administering haemodynamically active drugs.

An adequate blood pressure will produce 40–50 ml of urine every hour. A urinary catheter may be necessary to monitor urine output.

The cause of the arrest and its effects on the heart may be shown by a 12 lead electrocardiogram. Any subsequent changes can be related back to this early recording.

Gastric distension

Early attempts at mouth to mouth or bag valve mask ventilation may have introduced air into the stomach. An initially misplaced tracheal tube will do the same. Gastric distention provokes vomiting and is uncomfortable. It is usually necessary to insert a nasogastric tube.

Conclusions

It must be accepted that a commitment to treating cardiac arrest is a commitment to intensive care after resuscitation. The patient should be managed in an intensive care unit and is likely to need at least a short period of elective ventilation.

Further reading

Newburg LA. Cerebral resuscitation: advances and controversies. *Ann Emerg Med* 1984; **13**: 853–6.
White BC, Aust SD, Arford KE, Aronson LD. Brain injury by ischaemic anoxia: hypotheses extension–a tale of ions? *Ann Emerg Med* 1984; **13**: 862–7.
Niemann JT, Rosborough JP. Effects of acidaemic and sodium bicarbonate therapy in advanced cardiopulmonary resuscitation. *Ann Emerg Med* 1984; **13**: 781–4.
Safar P. Recent advances in cardiocerebral resuscitation: a review. *Ann Emerg Med* 1984; **13**: 856–62.
Redmond AD, Edwards JD. Haemodynamics during and after cardiac arrest. In: Vincent JL, ed. *Update in intensive care and emergency medicine*. Berlin: Springer, 1989; 531–8.
Cohn JN. Blood pressure measurement in shock. *JAMA* 1967; **199**: 972–6.

20 CARDIAC PACING AND RESUSCITATION

Michael C Colquhoun

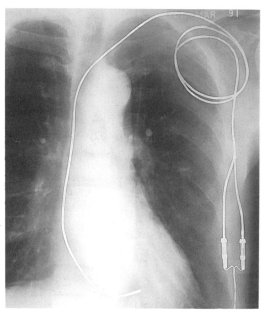

Chest radiograph showing temporary transvenous pacing system. Transvenous pacing is the method of choice for temporary pacing.

An artificial cardiac pacemaker is a device for administering an electrical current to the myocardium so that depolarisation and cardiac contraction occur. The earliest pacemakers were introduced in the 1950s and attempted to stimulate the heart by applying electrodes to the chest wall. Although effective, large currents were required and caused pain, skeletal muscle contraction, and burns to the skin.

Because of the problems with early external (or non-invasive) pacemakers, internal (or invasive) cardiac pacing was developed; the myocardium is stimulated directly by an electrode placed against the endocardium or epicardium. Epicardial pacing requires thoracotomy and has limited application; it is used for temporary pacing after cardiac surgery and occasionally when permanent pacing cannot be achieved by other means. Endocardial pacing, with an electrode introduced by the transvenous route, is now the usual method for both temporary and permanent pacing.

Recent technical advances have overcome many of the problems previously experienced with non-invasive (external) pacemakers, and modern external pacemakers offer a valuable method of achieving emergency cardiac pacing.

Indications for pacing

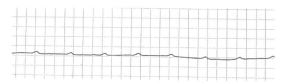

Ventricular standstill: P waves are seen but no QRS complexes. Pacing this should be considered in asystolic cardiac arrest when any electrical activity is present.

The principal indication for pacing is the treatment of bradycardia. Bradycardia may arise because of failure of the sinoatrial node to generate an impulse or because of subsequent block in conduction within the atrioventricular node or His-Purkinje system. Occasionally, problems in the sinoatrial node may be associated with more distal conduction problems in the same patient. Sinus arrest and more severe degrees of atrioventricular nodal block account for the implantation of the great majority of permanent pacemaker systems today. The same bradycardias may also be encountered during resuscitation attempts and require temporary pacing (see chapter 4).

It is important to remember that bradycardia or conduction disturbance may precede cardiac arrest and that their prompt recognition and treatment may prevent the subsequent arrest. This is particularly important in patients with acute myocardial infarction, when lesser degrees of conduction disturbance may precede the development of complete heart block; prophylactic pacing should be considered in these circumstances. Pacing should also be considered in the treatment of asystolic cardiac arrest when any electrical activity that may represent sporadic atrial or QRS complexes is present.

A second indication for pacing is in the treatment of tachycardias. In this setting a paced beat is used to interrupt the tachycardia and create an opportunity for sinus rhythm to become re-established. Atrial flutter and certain forms of junctional tachycardia may be converted to sinus rhythm by atrial pacing. Overdrive ventricular pacing has been used to treat certain refractory ventricular arrhythmias but requires the backup of a cardioverter defibrillator. In addition, some malignant ventricular arrhythmias may be prevented by accelerating the underlying heart rate by pacing; this is particularly true of the Torsade de Pointes type of polymorphic tachycardia.

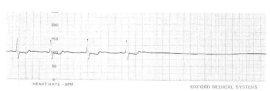

The onset of asystole; prophylactic pacing may prevent asystolic cardiac arrest.

Pacemakers

The pulse generator

All pacemakers consist of two basic components: a pulse generator and one or more pacing electrodes. The generator has a power source

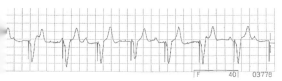

Ventricular pacing: a pacing spike precedes each QRS complex.

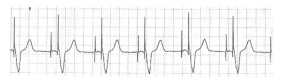

Dual chamber pacing: a pacing spike initiates both atrial and ventricular depolarisation.

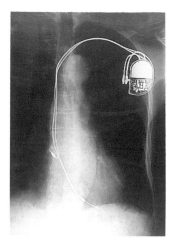

Permanent pacemaker with pacing electrodes in both atria and ventricle.

Pacing terminology

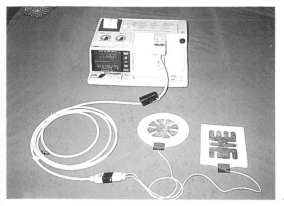

Non-invasive external pacemaker and electrodes.

and the electrical circuitry necessary to deliver the pacing stimuli. Temporary pacing units are relatively large and usually placed on the patient's bedside; a cable connects the unit to the pacing electrode inserted percutaneously into a vein. Controls enable the rate, sensitivity, and output to be controlled.

Permanent pacemakers are much smaller and are designed to be buried under the skin, usually in the upper thoracic region. Some modern units enable pacing of both the atria and ventricles sequentially to mimic the normal cardiac cycle, and some will automatically increase the pacing rate when there is a physiological demand for a faster heart rate.

The pacing stimulus

The discharge from the pacemaker arises almost instantaneously to the preset output voltage of the generator (usually about 5 volts) and then decays slowly over the course of 5 msec; after this it falls abruptly. The conventional electrocardiograph is not capable of following these rapid fluctuations, and in most cases the pacing stimulus (also known as the stimulus artifact) is seen as a single small spike. While this may not provide the detailed information required for pacemaker follow up, the recognition of the presence or absence of the stimulus artifact is often sufficient for analysis of the cardiac rhythm.

Pacing electrodes (wires, catheters, or leads)

With an endocardial pacemaking system two types of pacing electrode are used to convey the pacing stimulus to the endocardium; a unipolar electrode has the cathode at the distal end of the lead while the anode is provided by the outer case of the generator; a bipolar electrode incorporates both the anode (proximal) and cathode (distal) about 1 cm apart at the distal end of the lead; both lie in contact with endocardium. There is little to choose between the two types; the unipolar system is more sensitive to intrinsic cardiac activity but is also more susceptible to external electrical interference and skeletal muscle potentials.

Modern non-invasive (external) pacemakers use two large high impedance adhesive electrodes that are placed on the patient's chest. These are connected to the pulse generator by cables and usually serve the dual function of pacing and electrocardiographic monitoring.

Capture

If the pacing stimulus is adequate to generate an action potential that is conducted to the remainder of the myocardium, "capture" is said to occur. On the electrocardiogram, the pacing stimulus will be followed immediately by depolarisation of the paced cardiac chamber; in the case of ventricular pacing a QRS complex will follow the pacing spike. During ventricular pacing, ventricular depolarisation is initiated at an ectopic focus and the QRS complexes will be broad, resembling ventricular premature beats. As it is almost always the right ventricle that is paced the QRS complexes resemble those seen in left bundle branch block. For this reason no diagnoses that rely on morphological changes in the QRS complex (for example, infarction, ischaemia, or ventricular hypertrophy) can be made from the appearance of the paced QRS complexes.

Threshold

The ventricular threshold is the minimum output from the pacemaker generator (usually measured in volts) that results in ventricular capture. With a temporary pacemaker system the threshold is usually determined by gradually reducing the output voltage until failure of capture occurs at a "threshold" level. Many permanent

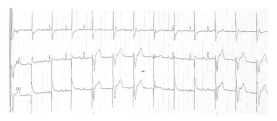

Fixed rate pacing.

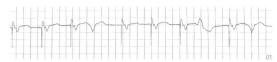

Demand pacing: the third, seventh, and ninth beats are spontaneous QRS complexes. These inhibit the pacemaker until the escape interval has elapsed when a further pacing stimulus is delivered.

pacemakers incorporate a program that allows the threshold to be measured non-invasively. When the program is activated the pacemaker gives a predetermined sequence of pacing stimuli of gradually decreasing strength. The threshold can be determined from the electrocardiogram by noting the point at which failure of capture occurs. With many of the more recent pacemakers, special equipment is required to activate this sequence, but with some older models the program can be activated with a magnet placed on the skin over the generator. Ideally, the ventricular threshold should lie between 0·5 and 1 volt, and the pacemaker output should be set to 5 volts or twice the threshold voltage in the case of a threshold of greater than 2·5 volts.

Fixed rate or asynchronous pacing

In this pacing mode the generator produces stimuli at regular intervals regardless of the underlying cardiac rhythm. Because competition between the paced beats and intrinsic rhythm may lead to serious ventricular arrhythmias this mode is rarely used.

Demand or synchronous pacing

With demand pacing the generator senses the intrinsic cardiac rhythm through the pacing electrode, and spontaneous complexes inhibit the output of the pacemaker. If the intrinsic heart rate is higher than the selected pacemaker rate, the generator will be inhibited completely. If, however, a spontaneous QRS complex is not followed by another one within an "escape" interval determined by the rate at which the pacemaker has been set, the pacemaker will generate an impulse. This minimises competition between natural and paced beats and reduces the risk of arrhythmias.

The demand mode is used in practically all pacemaking systems today. It must be remembered, however, that if a patient has two pacing systems (as may be the case where a temporary system has been inserted in a patient with a permanent system) the output of one generator may inhibit the other with complete loss of pacing. Careful selection or programming of the rates of the two systems may minimise competition, but it is often necessary to set the temporary system to the fixed rate mode to avoid inhibition by the output from the other generator.

Most permanent pacemakers will be converted from the demand mode to the fixed rate mode if a magnet is held over the generator. The "magnet rate" is usually about 90 impulses a minute and may reveal pacemaker function that is not evident when the spontaneous rhythm exceeds the demand rate.

Emergency cardiac pacing

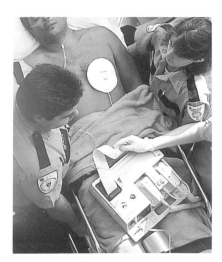

Emergency external pacing may be instituted outside hospital and will buy time until insertion of a transvenous system is possible.

Even when cardiac pacing is requried in an emergency there is often time to move the patient to a room where the catheter can be inserted under x ray screening control and in sterile conditions.

During resuscitation it will not usually be possible to move the patient and the necessary staff may not be rapidly available; this applies particularly outside hospital. It is under these circumstances that non-invasive external pacing can be used until the placement of a transvenous system is possible.

External pacing

Two adhesive electrodes are attached to the patient's chest, the cathode in a position corresponding to V3 of the electrocardiograph and the anode on the left posterior chest beneath the scapula. The electrodes are connected to the generator which is turned on to the selected rate, and the pacing current is increased until capture occurs. Pacing is achieved very rapidly without having to move the patient and without the need for x ray screening facilities. Because the technique is so easy to perform, pacing can be undertaken by many grades of staff. It is, however, a temporising measure and should be followed by the insertion of a temporary transvenous pacemaker as soon as circumstances allow.

Techniques designed to enable the placement of a transvenous pacing electrode without x ray screening, and the technique of transthoracic pacing (when a pacing electrode is inserted into the right ventricle through a percutaneous needle inserted through the chest wall) can no longer be recommended if non-invasive pacing is available.

Transvenous pacing

Route of venous access—In most cases the venous circulation will be entered by a central vein, either the subclavian or internal jugular. Various types of needles and introducers are available; the operator must be familiar with the one in use and follow the manufacturer's instructions. With central venous cannulation, manipulation of the pacing electrode is easier than when peripheral veins are used and the final position of the electrode is more stable. When the antecubital or femoral veins are used, limb movements greatly increase the risk of causing electrode displacement with potentially disastrous loss of pacing.

Aseptic technique—The pacing wire may have to remain in place for several days so full surgical aseptic techniques should be used by the operator to minimise the risk of infection. Once in place the catheter should be covered with a sterile dressing and the area should be inspected frequently for signs of phlebitis or sepsis.

Electrocardiographic monitoring—Throughout the procedure the electrocardiogram must be clearly visible to the operator. If the monitoring electrodes are not radiotranslucent they should be attached to the limbs rather than to the chest so that they do not obscure the picture on the image intensifier.

Other equipment—An intravenous cannula should be in place and other resuscitation equipment, including a defibrillator and drugs, must be available.

Pacing electrodes–The diameters used usually vary between 5F and 7F. The thinner 5F is more difficult for the beginner to manipulate, but the increased flexibility may enable the tricuspid valve to be crossed more easily. Being less stiff than the thicker wires, a 5F may also reduce the risk of perforating the right ventricle.

Technique—The catheter should be held between the thumbs and forefingers of both hands, well away from the entry point in the skin. It should be advanced, a few centimetres at a time, while maintaining its natural curve in line with the course of the major veins and vena cava; rotation of the catheter between thumb and forefinger may help. It can usually be advanced into the right atrium without difficulty and may easily cross the tricuspid valve to enter the right ventricle.

In cases of difficulty in entering the ventricle, the catheter should be "caught" on the lateral wall of the right atrium, formed into a loop, and then rotated; the loop will be seen suddenly to straighten out as the right ventricle is entered. Once in the ventricle, the electrode tip should be advanced to a stable position near the apex, and sufficient electrode should be advanced into the heart so that tip is not displaced by respiratory excursions or changes in posture.

The electrode should now be connected to the pacing generator and the threshold determined. If this is too high (above 1 volt) the electrode tip should be repositioned and the process repeated. A satisfactory threshold may sometimes be difficult to obtain, particularly when the ventricle is scarred or ischaemic. When satisfactorily positioned, stability of the catheter is checked by asking the patient to take a deep breath or cough while pacing the ventricle; any loss of capture indicates the need to reposition the electrode.

The heart should now be paced briefly at 10 volts to check for the absence of diaphragmatic stimulation. If these checks are satisfactory the pacemaker can be switched to the appropriate rate in demand mode.

The catheter should be secured to the skin near the point of entry by winding the skin suture material round it. Several loops of catheter should be formed to minimise the risk of displacement if the proximal catheter is pulled.

Finally, a chest *x* ray picture should be obtained to document electrode position and to exclude a pneumothorax or other complications.

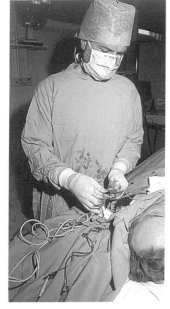

Insertion of a transvenous pacing system must be performed with aseptic surgical techniques.

Defibrillation

Special care is needed when performing defibrillation in a patient fitted with a cardiac pacemaker. Modern pacemakers are fitted with protection circuits that make it unlikely that the defibrillatory shock will damage the generator itself. Current may, however, travel down the pacing electrode and cause burns at the site where the electrode tip lies against the myocardium. This may lead to a rise in pacing threshold that may become apparent a considerable time after the shock; so if resuscitation is successful regular checks on the threshold should be carried out for two months.

To minimise the risk of damage to the pacemaker or electrode the defibrillator electrodes should be placed at least 12·5 cm from the generator when defibrillation is carried out. With temporary external pacemakers the electrodes or conductive gel must not be allowed to come into contact with the pacing wire or associated equipment.

The implantable cardioverter-defibrillator (ICD)

During the past decade implantable cardioverter defibrillators have been developed for the treatment of life threatening ventricular tachycardias. The pulse generator (which resembles a large pacemaker) is implanted beneath the skin and connected to a transvenous electrode placed endocardially in the heart. The device monitors the electrocardiogram through this electrode and recognises ventricular fibrillation or ventricular tachycardia at a rate above a predetermined level. Five to 10 seconds are required to recognise the arrhythmia and, after a charging period of about five seconds, a shock of up to 34 joules is delivered. The generators, which weigh between 200 and 300 g, are capable of delivering between 100 and 150 shocks during their lifespan of three to five years.

Patients successfully resuscitated from cardiac arrest who are at risk of further episodes or patients with recurrent ventricular arrhythmias resistant to other forms of treatment comprise the main groups of patients for whom this type of defibrillation is indicated.

The most recent models incorporate backup ventricular pacing facilities in case of bradycardia (as may follow defibrillation) and for antitachycardia pacing. They are capable of delivering tiered treatment: ventricular extrastimulus; cardioversion at 3 joules; and defibrillation at 3–34 joules.

Further reading

Bennett DH. Management of bradycardias. In: Julian DG, et al, eds. *Diseases of the heart*. London: Baillière Tindall, 1989.

Crockett P, McHugh LG. Non-invasive pacing—what you should know. Physio Control Corporation, 1988. (Tel 01256 474455).

INDEX

Index

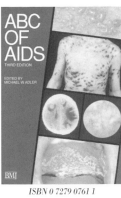
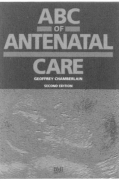
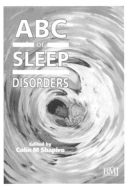
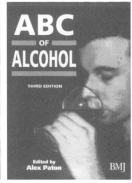
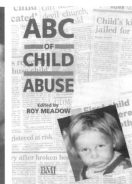
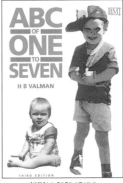
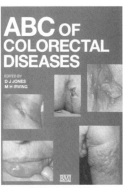
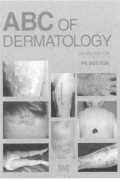
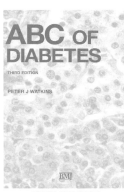
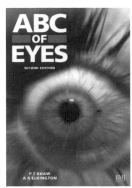
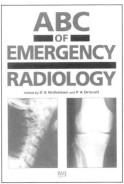
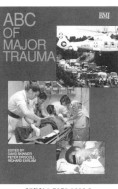
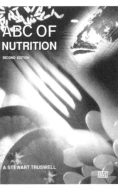
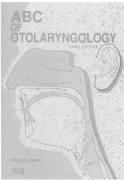
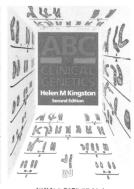
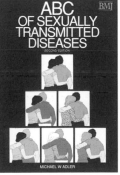
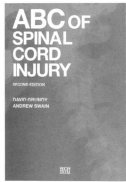
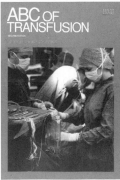
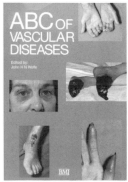
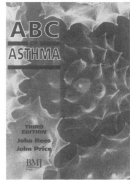
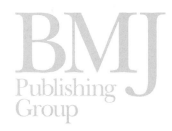